Integrative Arts Psychotherapy

This book is a new addition to the art therapy literature setting out an integrative approach to using theory and the arts, which places clients at the centre of practice and supports collaboration across the therapeutic journey. The structural framework described enables different theories, contemporary research, and best-practice guidelines to be used to inform therapy, allowing the practitioner to work fluidly and rigorously in response to their clients' changing needs and therapeutic aims.

Integrative arts psychotherapy brings therapeutic practice to life, as the use of the visual arts is enhanced by the possibilities offered for developing and deepening therapeutic work using sculpture/clay, drama/puppetry, poetry, sand play, music, and bodywork/movement. The work described in this book has grown from a British and European art therapy culture, community, and history – influenced by prominent American theorists.

The book has been written for trainers, trainees, and practitioners of creative arts therapies, psychotherapy, and expressive arts therapies – nationally and worldwide. It may also be of interest to other professionals, or those in consultation with an art therapist, who want to understand what this type of art therapy can offer.

Claire Louise Vaculik (née Leyland) is an HCPC-registered art therapist and UKCP-registered Gestalt psychotherapist. She is Programme Director of the MA in Integrative Arts Psychotherapy at the Institute for Arts in Therapy and Education and Chair of the British Association of Art Therapists.

Gary Nash, Dip AT, MAAT, is an HCPC-registered art therapist. Gary co-founded the London Art Therapy Centre in 2009, where he is a practitioner-researcher. He is a visiting lecturer at the Institute for Arts in Therapy and Education and the University of Hertfordshire. He is a co-editor of *Environmental Arts Therapy* (2020).

Integrative Arts Psychotherapy

Using an Integrative Theoretical Frame and the Arts in Psychotherapy

Edited by Claire Louise Vaculik and Gary Nash

Routledge
Taylor & Francis Group

LONDON AND NEW YORK

Cover image: Man. Oil on canvas. 24 x 20 inches by Emma Cameron.

First published 2022
by Routledge
4 Park Square, Milton Park, Abingdon, Oxon OX14 4RN

and by Routledge
605 Third Avenue, New York, NY 10158

Routledge is an imprint of the Taylor & Francis Group, an informa business

British Library Cataloguing-in-Publication Data
A catalogue record for this book is available from the British Library

Library of Congress Cataloging-in-Publication Data
A catalog record for this book has been requested

ISBN: 978-0-367-72637-9 (hbk)
ISBN: 978-0-367-72636-2 (pbk)
ISBN: 978-1-003-15567-6 (ebk)

DOI: 10.4324/9781003155676

Typeset in Times New Roman
by Apex CoVantage, LLC

We would like to dedicate this book to Dr Ken Pickering and Professor Maria Gilbert, who played such an important role in the development of integrative arts psychotherapy. They are both much missed.

Contents

Illustrations

Diagram

Figures

Biographies

Claire Louise Vaculik (née Leyland) is the current Chair of the British Association of Art Therapists (BAAT). She is an HCPC-registered art therapist (Goldsmiths) and UKCP-registered Gestalt psychotherapist (Metanoia Institute). Since 2009, she has been the Programme Director of the MA in Integrative Arts Psychotherapy at the Institute for Arts in Therapy and Education (IATE), training integrative arts psychotherapists. Claire Louise was, until recently, an External Examiner of the MA in Art Therapy programme – at both the University of Chester and at the University of Derby – and a Lead Assessor on the Assessment Board of the UKCPs Humanistic and Integrative College. From 2008–2014, Claire Louise was an Associate Editor of the *International Journal of Art Therapy: Inscape*, working with authors and reviewers to develop submissions for the art therapy journal. In her clinical practice, she has worked extensively with both children and adults in hospices, bereavement services and in education, using a trauma-informed approach. She ran a service that supports children, young people, and staff in schools and sees clients in private practice.

Gary Nash, Dip AT, MAAT, is an HCPC-registered art therapist who trained in 1989 and 1995 at both Goldsmiths' and St Albans College of Art. He has developed a private practice since 1995 alongside his work in social services, the voluntary sector, and mainstream education. He was Co-Founder of the London Art Therapy Centre in 2009, where he is a practitioner-researcher providing individual and group arts psychotherapy and delivering professional workshops and training for art therapists and leading on arts-based research. He also established the BAAT Special Interest Group in Private Practice in 2010, which provides a professional forum for art therapists working in private practice. He is a visiting lecturer at IATE and the University of Hertfordshire and co-editor of Environmental arts therapy, Routledge, 2020.

Chapter authors

Dr Marie Adams is a writer and psychotherapist with a private practice in Dorset. Initially trained as Person-Centred Counsellor, she then continued training in integrative and psychoanalytic therapy. She is an academic advisor and module leader on the DPsych programme at Metanoia and also teaches at IATE (University of East London), based in Islington. A former journalist with the BBC, she has a research interest in how therapists' personal lives impact their work. Her book, *The Myth of the Untroubled Therapist (2014)* is a standard text on counselling and psychotherapy courses throughout the country. She is also the author of the novel, *Telling Time (2015)*, and has written extensively on creativity in academic writing. While Marie has a particular interest in therapists and creative writing, her current academic research is focused on the somatic aspects of research writing.

Marrianne Behm is an arts psychotherapist, supervisor, and lecturer with over 20 years experience in clinical settings in both adolescent and adult mental health. She is the Head Arts Psychotherapist at an inner-city National Health Service (NHS) Foundation Trust. Her department focuses on psychotic, mood and personality disorders and trauma. Marrianne has a private practice in central London as well as an online service for both supervision and personal therapy. She is a lecturer and tutor on the MA Integrative Arts psychotherapy course at IATE and also teaches on their Post Graduate Certificate in the Therapeutic Arts. Marrianne trained in art psychotherapy at Goldsmiths and now combines a psychodynamic approach with integrative models. She has also trained in the use of a variety of approaches, including Mentalization Based Treatment (MBT) and Trauma Informed approach, and the use of sand play. Marrianne is also a practicing artist.

Graeme Blench, LLCMTD, Dip MUSIC THERAPY, Dip SD, is a qualified music therapist and psychotherapist. Graeme has taught at IATE since 1987. He is Head of Staff and Students, and he sits on the Senior Management Committee and Academic Board. His specialist areas are music therapy, transactional analysis, Gestalt, group dynamics, and psychodynamic theory and practice.

Anthea Benjamin, MAIAP, is a UKCP- and BACP-registered Integrative Arts Psychotherapist, Adolescent Psychotherapist, Certified DDP Practitioner, Clay Field Therapist, Play Therapist, Group Analyst, Trainer, Supervisor, and Organisational Consultant. Anthea has worked extensively with children, adolescents, adults, families, couples, and groups for over 18 years in various settings including schools, community projects, within the NHS, and her private practice. Anthea works as a therapist delivering training and consultancy in a range of professional and educational contexts. Anthea also offers therapeutic services such as self-reflective groups and team supervision, both in organisations with a particular focus on culture change. Anthea has a special interest in racial trauma, particularly working with racial trauma in the body.

Emma Cameron, Dip IAP, MAIAP, is an established artist, HCPC- and UKCP-registered integrative arts psychotherapist, and clinical supervisor, who has been in private practice in north Essex since 2014. She has been working with clients online since 2016. An ACTO member with diplomas in online therapy and online supervision, she has delivered training on online practice to art therapy training institutions and professional organisations in the UK and Ireland. Since 2018, Emma has also been incorporating Accelerated Experiential Dynamic Psychotherapy (AEDP) into her practice. Emma's website features an extensive range of her articles, podcast interviews, and resources on a range of therapy-related topics. Emma is part of the staff teams at IATE in London, and Matrix College in Norfolk.

Jack Eastwood, MA in dramatherapy, is a dramatherapist and storyteller. He has been working in psychiatric inpatient care in the NHS for the past 15 years. He supervises and mentors younger therapists, works in private practice, and teaches meditation. Along with psychotherapists and puppeteers from *The River of Soul*, he leads workshops and week-long retreats exploring myths and stories for therapeutic learning. Jack's earlier career was as a performer in a three-man troupe, which toured the world for 18 years. Known as *The Moving Picture Mime Show*, they created high-energy mask and movement theatre – a modern take on the commedia dell'arte. He originally trained with Jacques Lecoq in Paris, and later trained in the Sesame approach to drama and movement therapy at London's Central School of Speech and Drama. He's a member of the British Association of Dramatherapists and registered with HCPC.

Sarah Hall is a Psychoanalytic Art Psychotherapist (UKCP, HCPC) and Jungian Analyst (BPC, IAAP) in Private Practice in Cornwall. She also works part time as clinical lead in dual diagnosis at Chy rehab in Truro and has taught on the MA Art Psychotherapy training at IATE, and currently teaches for the Society of Social and Critical Psychoanalysis. As a professional artist and former academic lecturer at Glasgow School of Art, she has been involved in researching the collective as well as personal impact of creativity by working in prisons, long stay hospitals and institutions. Her current PhD research involves a Jungian interpretation of drug dreams in patients in recovery from addiction and the implications for clinical practice.

Tsafi Lederman is an Integrative Arts Psychotherapist, Gestalt, and Body Psychotherapist who specialises in integrating body processes with the arts in psychotherapy. She runs a private psychotherapy, a supervision practice and has been a trainer, working with individuals and groups, for over 30 years. Tsafi is a senior lecturer and tutor on the Diploma and MA in Integrative Arts Psychotherapy. She was Co-Director of the MA in Creativity and Imagination at IATE. Originally, Tsafi graduated from art school and studied expressive movement and theatre in Japan. She has contributed to chapters and articles in the area of therapeutic relationship in clinical work for psychotherapists, physical therapists, and coaches.

Dr Vanja Orlans is a Director of Psychology Matters Ltd. In her work, she helps individuals, groups, and organisations to reflect on and implement change through approaches that include psychotherapy, group work, teaching, and consultancy. She was formerly a Faculty Head at Metanoia Institute in London and Programme Leader of the Doctorate in Counselling Psychology and Psychotherapy by Professional Studies (DCPsych), a joint programme with Middlesex University. She is a British Psychological Society (BPS) Chartered Psychologist and is registered with the HCPC as both a Counselling Psychologist and an Occupational Psychologist. She is also a UKCP-registered Gestalt Psychotherapist and Senior Practitioner Member of the BPS Register of Psychologists Specialising in Psychotherapy. Vanja has published widely in the fields of psychology and psychotherapy and is the co-author of *Integrative Therapy: 100 Key Points and Techniques* published by Routledge. She teaches and practises in London.

Hannah Rees, MSc Gestalt Psychotherapy, has been a UKCP-registered Gestalt psychotherapist, clinical supervisor, and EMDR practitioner in private practice since 2007. She has a background in classical singing and running Natural Voice workshops. She specialises in a trauma-informed and body-centred approach including voicework which she calls improvised dyadic singing. She currently supervises at the Women and Girls Network and Jewish Women's Aid. Previously she was the clinical lead at North London Rape Crisis. Her work at Portsmouth Abuse and Rape Centre was subject to a research project that inspired the illustrated book, *The Courage to be Me*, by Dr Nina Burrowes.

Daniel Regan is a photographic artist specialising in complex and difficult emotional experiences, focusing on the transformational impact of arts on mental health, building on his own lived experience. As part of his practice, Daniel also shoots commissions, runs socially engaged projects, and provides consultancy. He regularly exhibits and speaks at events across fine art, educational, and clinical institutions in the UK and worldwide. Daniel is Executive Director of the Arts & Health Hub, a not-for-profit organisation that supports artists that work in the arts and health sector. Previously, he was Artistic Director of a pioneering arts and health organisation within the NHS.

Rebecca Smart, MAIAP, is an HCPC- and UKCP-registered Integrative Arts Psychotherapist (IATE). She is Lead Arts Psychotherapist for Wiltshire, AWP NHS Trust, managing an arts psychotherapies team and offering clinical supervision, consultation, and reflective practice groups for staff. Her NHS clinical work is based in the community, where she specialises in working with complex trauma. Rebecca has trained in EMDR and Internal Family Systems Therapy, which she integrates into her work. She has a private practice and is also a storyteller and ecotherapist, offering groups in the woods exploring myth and creative process. Rebecca has trained in Embodied Systemic Coaching and Constellations (ICF cert.) and has a background as a facilitator and coach specialising in communication, storytelling, resilience, organisational change, and leadership development, for a diverse range of global organisations. Rebecca is an Academic Advisor and Marker for the MA programme at IATE.

Jude Smit is a UKCP- and HCPC-registered Psychotherapist/Integrative Arts Psychotherapist, working with groups and individuals in a range of settings, including a hospital, Further and Higher Education, and private practice. She has a special interest in trauma and has completed training in various trauma treatment protocols, including EMDR. Jude is Deputy Programme Director for the MA in Integrative Arts Psychotherapy at IATE. Over the last 18 years, Jude has been involved in various research projects focused on mental health, within the education and health sectors, and has presented at conferences internationally. She is currently completing Psychology PhD research, focusing on students' lived experiences of attempted suicide.

Dr Margot Sunderland is a Founding Director of IATE, a Higher Education College. The Institute offers Masters' Degree courses in Integrative Arts Psychotherapy, Integrative Child Psychotherapy, and many other related courses in child counselling and therapeutic play. She is also Director of Education and Training at the Centre for Child Mental Health London, Co-Director of Trauma Informed Schools UK, an Honorary Visiting Fellow at London Metropolitan University, and child psychotherapist with over 30 years of experience in working with children and teenagers. Dr Sunderland is the author of over 20 books, which collectively have been translated into 18 languages and published in 24 countries. Her internationally acclaimed book, *What Every Parent Needs to Know*, endorsed by world-leading neuroscientist Professor Jaak Panksepp, won First Prize in the British Medical Association Medical Book awards 2007 (Popular Medicine section). The book has also been voted one of the top brain books of our time by The Dana Foundation. Dr Sunderland undertakes many speaking engagements on her work in the UK and abroad.

Acknowledgements

We would like to start at the beginning by acknowledging the individuals who have shown us what worked for them in therapy. Whether calling themselves clients, service users, or patients, they have always been equal partners in the therapeutic relationship. These unique people have each helped us to learn and understand how to integrate and move between art forms, so that we can meet their experiences and needs creatively, and imaginatively, in an art form that speaks to them.

We would like to express our special thanks and gratitude to the students and graduates of the MA in Integrative Arts Psychotherapy course at IATE. It has been an honour to be part of your learning journey. We have been touched and inspired by the passion, bravery, creativity, and commitment that you have shown on this path, as you have worked to be present with and support each of your clients in the manner that most enables their growth.

Also, to the teaching, administrative, and operations staff teams at IATE, who work so hard to provide a caring, vibrant, and nurturing foundation from which students can learn, explore, question, and then continue to develop integrative arts psychotherapy practice on their ongoing professional journeys.

Foreword

Therapeutic communities of creation

Shaun McNiff

In the early 1970s when I established the first graduate programme to integrate all forms of artistic expression in education and therapy, there were strong forces in favour of relaxing boundaries between professions and academic fields. We were supported by the Commonwealth of Massachusetts Department of Mental Health, which was implementing comprehensive multidisciplinary training to further community-based practice. To minimise fragmentation, the arts in therapy disciplines were asked to consolidate and work together alongside medicine, psychology, and social work (McNiff, 2009, pp. 23, 255). We embraced the initiative and offered comprehensive arts therapy services while maintaining the integrity of individual art forms. The programme was well received by mental health and education sites, locally and internationally, and in a short time, we enrolled students from throughout the world.

For decades beginning in the early 1980s, I was immersed in supporting the development of the arts in therapy within continental Europe. Other than transit stops at Heathrow, I had little contact with the UK art therapy community. In 2009, Ross Prior then at the University of Northampton invited me to address the international conference that led to his founding of the Journal of Applied Arts and Health. When IATE heard that I would be in the country, I was asked to offer a daylong studio session. I was taken aback by the IATE community – the passionate and open-minded participants, the commitment to various forms of artistic expression, and the physical structure of the art space created in a former commercial building on London's Britannia Row. I felt a complete congruence with my commitment to *whole art expression* as supported by the Institute's studio environment. In the arts therapies, we often work in difficult spaces, usually not constructed to support art making, and rarely conducive to the full spectrum of expressive possibilities as I experienced at IATE.

The visit led to close collaboration with the UK and return trips to England. In 2018 while working with Gary Nash and the team at the London Art Therapy Centre, I met Claire Louise Vaculik. We spoke about the history of IATE and its unique embrace of all art forms within the UK community. Where the many integrated arts therapy programmes and training centres in continental Europe, the Middle East, Asia, and the Americas have ties to our initiatives in the United States, I was fascinated with how IATE originated independently with no direct contact. The same applied to the "multi-arts/multimodal" approaches in Melbourne, Australia, in the 1990s, developed first at La Trobe University and then at the Melbourne Institute for Experiential and Creative Arts Therapies (MIECAT) founded in 1997. As with IATE, the MIECAT programme with its emphasis on transdisciplinary and experiential learning took shape outside the established structures of higher education. In the Southern Hemisphere, the integration of the arts extended to New Zealand, where Sylvia Ashton-Warner and Elwyn Richardson earlier made classic contributions, with the establishment of the graduate programme in Creative Arts Therapy at Whitecliffe College. Warren Lett (1936–2019), the founding director of MIECAT, published various accounts of the community's focus on collaborative and practice-centred enquiry in what they describe as a "companioning" process (Lett, 2016). In 2021, I guest-edited a special issue of the *Journal of Applied Arts in Health* reflecting on the contributions that Warren made to our international community (2021b, 2021c) and I am grateful to continue the reflections on origins and shared visions in relation to IATE.

During our work together in London, I urged Claire Louise and Gary to create a book documenting the history and methods of IATE. In addition to making the international community aware of the formative work being done in England, I felt that the publication would further understanding of the autonomous development of integrated arts programmes in different sectors of the world, all designed to respond to the unique needs and interests of individual persons and groups.

When first introduced to IATE, I was eager to learn about the processes informing the creation of its unique approach within the larger and more specialised arts in psychotherapy community of the UK. I was told that the institution grew from the work of Margot Sunderland with young people in the mid-1980s. When I received the manuscript for this book, I read with great interest how the IATE mission emerged. Margot describes how in her collaboration with Dr Ken Pickering and Dr Stephen Little, they determined that an exclusive focus on only one art form would limit their ability to enhance "self-expression, self-exploration, and healing". As in my experience, they considered how access to various forms of artistic expression might enable creative processes to manifest themselves more completely and respond to individual preferences and needs.

I was surprised to learn that Malcolm Ross had a significant role in the founding of IATE and the development of its first graduate degree programme in cooperation with the University of Exeter. After collaborating with Malcolm at two international conferences organised by Ross Prior at the University of Wolverhampton, the most recent focusing on "Building Bridges" amongst health professions, and not yet knowing of his formative connections to IATE, I said to myself, "This explains everything – 'Six degrees of separation'". Malcolm's ability to respond to the present moments of the creative process spontaneously and authentically with contextually sensitive expressions perfectly fits the objectives of total art expression (*Gesamtkunstwerk*). Margot tells how she was influenced by Malcolm's work as the founding chair of the UK's National Association for the Arts in Education and his writings, including *The Aesthetic Impulse* (1984).

When forming IATE, Margot, Ken, and Stephen decided that they would combine therapy and education training through an integrative process to expand and reach more people in diverse settings. This assimilation of therapy and education characterised the graduate programmes at the Institute for the Arts and Human Development at Lesley College (now Lesley University) in Cambridge, Massachusetts, that I established in the early 1970s. The two most influential faculty members in relation to furthering the development of arts integration in therapy, Norma Canner and Paolo Knill, were then teaching in the Eliot Pearson Department of Child Study and Human Development at nearby Tufts University. In early childhood education, inspired by infant schools in the UK, fluidity of expression was pervasive. Norma, who had a background in theatre as well as dance, taught us all how to work with large groups and communities. Paolo, based at the Winterthur Conservatory in Switzerland, was applying the psychology of Jean Piaget to music. He became my closest partner and committed his career to researching the process of arts integration in therapy with significant international impact. And interestingly, in researching the history of Warren Lett's work in Melbourne, I discovered that he began his career as a teacher before concentrating on counselling and psychotherapy. His approach to the use of artistic enquiry in therapy, education, and other professions has been sustained by the MIECAT mission.

We might ask: what is it about education, or education in the period of the 1960s and 1970s, that fostered this progressive and integral approach to therapy and artistic expression? Is it as likely to happen today when there is arguably less emphasis on the interrelatedness of all modes of learning and creative expression?

Maxwell Jones (1907–1990), who pioneered the therapeutic community movement, originally in the UK (Jones, 1968), regretted in his last years that there was a regression away from open, practical, and creative change in mental health. In 1970, I was introduced to his work by my group therapy supervisor at a large Massachusetts state hospital. In the early 1980s, I established a relationship with Max based on our common thinking about the creative process, community, and problems with reductionistic psychology, and in 1985, he invited me to address the annual meeting of the American Association of Social Psychiatry. We explored how egalitarian approaches to "open systems" (Jones, 1982) and his growing interest in social ecology were closely aligned with my group studios that I have called therapeutic communities of creation based upon the interdependence of all forms of artistic expression. Those of us interested in a depth psychology of art and therapy, and especially when inviting the full spectrum of imaginative possibilities, might consider how our empirical practice is a manifestation of nature's eco-systems of creation that hold all of life (McNiff, 2021a).

In studying the origins of the various places from which integration and transdisciplinary cooperation took shape in the arts therapies, they were all grounded in both therapy and education while generating strong values of collaboration spanning academic and professional silos with the goal of affirming diverse experiences, interests, roles, and abilities. There was a realisation that artistic expressions can take infinitely different forms while also sharing common features. All the programmes were characterised by an overriding commitment to a supportive community of practice. During my admission interviews with students from throughout the world in the 1970s and 1980s, they described an unrealised need to create within environments supporting their various artistic passions. To the extent that integrated approaches were different from the norm, and often at odds with dominant systems, this increased a sense of purpose amongst us.

The authors similarly describe opposition from specialised disciplines, stated perfectly in the first lines of their Introduction. The process is archetypal, manifesting consistent dynamics, invariably related to power, control, and the protection of financial, "territorial", and "organisational" interests rather than cooperation based on "shared" principles, together with sincere differences as to what constitutes quality practice. The same tensions have existed for generations in relation to specialised and liberal education with the latter perceiving all things as interconnected with depth requiring breadth.

The case against integration and breadth characteristically emphasises the purported dangers of insufficient training and competency, and how the absence of credentials in a specific art form dangerously promotes Jacks (or Jacquelines) of all trades and impostors, the dilution of quality, and so forth. The accusation that the integrity of art forms is compromised by integration is false. I have only observed full commitment to the pursuit of excellence in all aspects of expression which is arguably improved rather than diminished by an embrace of the fullness of persons and artistic processes. In my experience, the integral approach has resulted in attracting outstanding practicing artists as both faculty and students. The sometimes "fierce" protection of borders as described here is not restricted to the UK. For me, the antagonisms have been beneficial, fuelling commitment and advocacy for a more inclusive, imaginative, and deeply authentic, art experience.

On the basis of my largely positive history in dealing with these issues, the most effective way of advancing values and methods that might differ from dominant paradigms is to articulate, demonstrate, and publish positions in sync with accepted principles of therapeutic practice and human experience – and most importantly, present the art evidence as convincingly as possible and let it speak for itself (McNiff, in press) as demonstrated in this book. As an advocate for the most comprehensive and accessible approaches to art and public health, my experience reliably affirms that artistic expression can be viewed as a force of nature, innate to people everywhere, and as accessible as breath (McNiff, 2015). If you can move, you can paint, draw, dance, perform, and create in various other media. Domains of art cannot be categorically fenced since expression will always fly over the enclosures which are themselves institutional constructs which can sometimes go against the grain of nature. Arguably, the primary deterrent to universal access is the specialised industries of artistic expression and their accompanying notions of talent which do more, worldwide, to exclude rather than include and inspire participation. In contrast, I encourage the close study of children's art, especially in the early years, before social inhibitions and judgements take hold. Of course, exceptional media skills are necessary for many sectors of artistic and professional practice. But this does not always apply to art and well-being where arguments for the most inclusive and comprehensive opportunities can be made.

Consider the concept of "art" which includes all forms of artistic expression made by artists in various disciplines from the violin, sculpture, ballet, theatre, filmmaking, and so forth. I have always been comfortable with the term art therapy, albeit I define it differently. The circumscribed institution of "art therapy", which is in fact "visual art therapy", has within itself endless forms of artistic expression. If we logically follow the rationale that the use of specific media of expression in therapy requires credentialing, should we begin to restrict the practice of those who introduce clay sculpture, print making, drawing, or digital media, respectively, to even more specialised disciplines? The arguments might be even stronger regarding music therapy where differences between instruments can be significant and where all are distinct from the voice which has grown significantly as a psychotherapeutic medium outside the music and drama therapy areas. The same applies to performance being larger than drama, and the body is not limited to dance. Within the narrowest of specialisations, there are numerous media and methods, and thus the potential credentialing can go into infinity.

When I wrote the book *Art-Based Research* (1998), I had the freedom to use the term for all forms of artistic expression because it was not tied to an organisational trademark. Simply stated, the arts therapy specialisations are extensions of institutions and not the organic making of art with its infinite variations. In keeping with the larger and more established professions of medicine and law, specialisations, often quite narrow, occur within them rather than becoming professions in themselves. While respecting a person's choice to pursue the most circumscribed artistic practices in therapy, I oppose making them into professions that control access.

Having the opportunity to work closely over the years with thousands of arts therapists from throughout the world, I can say categorically that the media skills of people in the highly specialised disciplines of art, dance, drama, music, and poetry therapy are not necessarily superior to those in expressive arts therapy, the trademark used to professionally designate those who work with more than one art form. And similarly, there are numerous examples throughout history of more generally credentialed therapists in areas such as psychiatry, who not only pioneered the use of artistic expression but also made significant art themselves – perhaps best exemplified by C. G. Jung, who anticipated just about everything we do with the arts in therapy and art-based research, with excellence, over 100 years ago.

If a person is dedicating a career to the use of art in therapy, the highest degree of media understanding will reliably be pursued – and clearly, some art forms require advanced skills and may be less accessible in certain situations. But most invite universal participation without compromising quality (McNiff, 2018). For example, my experience encouraging the movement basis of art making suggests that our elemental gestures inherently strive for the most effective expression (McNiff, 2015).

In relation to arts therapy training, I say: perfect your various disciplines so that in addition to professional practice, you can lead, supervise, and foster the most comprehensive public access, as well as the participation of artists, educators, health professionals, and volunteers – but do not use your credential to limit participation. Strong support for the credentialing of therapists does not necessarily extend to the infinite forms of communication and creation that they might use, modes of expression with inherent healing properties which must be universally accessible (McNiff, 2004).

Finally, as someone who does not identify with a particular "school" of therapeutic practice other than how art heals by engaging difficulties and transforming them into affirmations of life while infusing persons and communities with creative energy, I want to wholeheartedly support this book's focus on integrative arts psychotherapy. As I say to students, I urge you to create your own methods of practice. If you critically study what I do, fine. But please do the work your way, based on your experience and place in the world. I urge the same with communities of practice in keeping with what I have said here about my fascination with the development of independent centres of arts integration throughout the world. My hope for the future is that this diversity of creations will grow and discourage stock methods of practice which are contrary to the nature of art. For example, in developing arts integration in therapy, our intention was never to develop methods that always move from one form of artistic expression to another, which is of course something that often happens when appropriate to given situations, wonderfully described in this book as "shapeshifting". The discipline in my view simply supports the use of more than one art form in relation to needs. When we paint, we may exclusively and seriously paint, and the same goes for dance, poetry, percussion, and so forth.

If a training programme dealing with the integration of the arts in therapy is going to organise itself according to a particular theory of practice, what could be more appropriate than this book's emphasis on integrating all the arts, the whole of life, and psychotherapeutic methods, and with a primary focus on the sanctity and primacy of therapeutic relationships coupled with a sensitivity to context?

Writing this Foreword has been an unexpected work of personal, artistic, and professional integration, inspired by a book that I trust will flourish within the context of its "relationships" with readers. The process has renewed my long-standing identification with the integral basis of life and human understanding. When John Norcross, now a leading figure in integrative psychotherapy and psychotherapy research, invited me in the mid-1980s to write about my work integrating the arts in therapy as a manifestation of integrative psychotherapy for a journal he was editing at the beginning of his distinguished career, I was impressed with the emphasis on the logical need for common-sense and practical approaches within a profession permeated by ideological separations. And regarding the use of art in therapy, the first line of my essay was: "Integrative psychotherapy can be perceived as an affirmation of the psyche's multiplicity and its varied modes of expression" (McNiff, 1987, p. 259). The case for an integrative framework has since made exponential gains throughout the world. My hope for the future is that it stays open to art's infinite uniqueness and methods of practice in various communities of creation.

Shaun McNiff, Gloucester, Massachusetts,
December 2021

Shaun McNiff's books and essays have been widely influential and translated into many languages. He leads art studios, lectures, and teaches throughout the world. Honors and awards include the Lifetime Achievement Award of the Journal of Applied Arts and Health and the Honorary Life Member Award of the American Art Therapy Association. McNiff was appointed as the first university professor at Lesley University in 2002. In 1974, he established the integrated arts therapy graduate training program at Lesley, from which the discipline of Expressive Arts Therapy emerged. He is an exhibiting painter who wrote the first book on art-based research and uses his ongoing artistic practice as the foundation for his work with others.

References

Jones, M. (1968). *Beyond the therapeutic community: Social learning and social psychiatry*. New Haven, CT: Yale University Press.

Jones, M. (1982). *The process of change*. Boston, London, Melbourne and Henley: Routledge & Kegan Paul.

Lett, W. (2016). *Creative arts companioning in coconstruction of meanings*. Melbourne: Warren Lett.

McNiff, S. (1987). Pantheon of creative arts therapies: An integrative perspective. *Journal of Integrative and Eclectic Psychotherapy*, 6(3), 259–281.

McNiff, S. (1998). *Art-based research*. London: Jessica Kingsley Publisher.

McNiff, S. (2004). *Art heals: How creativity cures the soul*. Boston: Shambhala Publications.

McNiff, S. (2009). *Integrating the arts in therapy: History, theory, and practice*. Springfield, IL: Charles C Thomas.

McNiff, S. (2015). *Imagination in action: Secrets for unleashing creative expression*. Boston: Shambhala Publications.

McNiff, S. (2018). All inclusive art making. *NiTRO – Non Traditional Research Outcomes, a Publication of the Australian Council of Deans and Directors of Creative Arts*, May 30. https://nitro.edu.au/articles/2018/5/30/all-inclusive-art-making

McNiff, S. (2021a). Revisioning art and nature: Toward a depth psychology of creation. *Ecopoiesis: Eco-Human Theory and Practice*, 2(1), 49–56 [open access internet journal] https://en.ecopoiesis.ru/articles/article_post/mcniff-shaun-revisioning-art-and-nature-toward-a-depth-psychology-of-creation

McNiff, S. (2021b). Introduction to the special section honouring Warren R. Lett. *The Journal of Applied Arts and Health*, 12(1), 9–5.

McNiff, S. (2021c). Companioning' in artistic inquiry: The practice & vision of Warren Lett (1935–2019) & the role of personal process in research. *Journal of Applied Arts and Health*, 12(1), 45–55.

McNiff, S. (in press). Art is the evidence: Convincing public communication of art-based research and its outcomes. In R. W. Prior, M. Kossak, & T. A. Fisher (Eds.), *Applied arts and health, education and community: Building bridges*. Bristol: Intellect and University of Chicago Press.

Ross, M. (1984). *The aesthetic impulse*. Oxford and New York: Pergamon Press.

Introduction to integrative arts psychotherapy

Claire Louise Vaculik and Gary Nash

Integrative arts psychotherapy: An historical perspective

The pioneering artists, teachers, and activists of the early 1960s were driven by a guiding principle of creative and political action. The formal organisation of what was then a marginalised group of artists and art teachers with a special interest in the remedial use of the arts in special education and psychiatric hospital settings led to the formation of the British Association of Art Therapists (BAAT) in 1964 (Waller, 1991, p. xii). Although there was no recognised training until 1971, between 1965 and 1971 the BAAT training sub-committee began to have discussions to examine the potential of designing an "arts therapy course" that included the use of art, movement and dance, and drama therapy. There were four reasons why this inspired vision did not happen: economic, structural, organisational, and territorial (Waller, 1991, p. 227). An integrative course would require cooperation between different arts departments, there were questions around which discipline would dominate and control the course identity, and there were also concerns around the need to have a clear definition for a pioneering new course at a time of cutbacks in education.

The first specialist art therapy certificate course was launched by John Evans and Edward Adamson at the St Albans School of Art, later Hertfordshire College of Art and Design in 1971, with the first Diploma in Art Therapy being validated by the Council for National Academic Awards in 1975. In the 1980s, the introduction of drama therapy and the dance movement therapy programmes at St Albans ushered in a 20-year period of mixed discipline teaching across the different arts therapies specialisms. This approach to parallel teaching on the arts therapies training at the master's level has continued at several current trainings, where students in visual arts, drama, music, and play therapy study alongside on some shared modules. The emergence of the integrative arts psychotherapy training at the Institute of Art in Therapy and Education (IATE) in 1986 is therefore unique in using the visual arts as a shared language whilst teaching the integration of all the arts within one multi-arts curriculum. Chapter 1 traces the formation, history, vision, and development of the MA in Integrative Arts Psychotherapy, the only course of its kind in Britain.

DOI: 10.4324/9781003155676-1

In Chapter 2, an art psychotherapist service manager describes how an NHS arts psychotherapy service developed to use an integrative arts approach over a 25-year timeframe, influenced by wider changes in health and psychological therapies and inspired, in part, by the work being done and taught at IATE.

Integrating the arts and relationship

Integrative psychotherapy is described by Gilbert and Orlans (2011) as using: "a unifying approach that brings together physiological, affective, cognitive, contextual and behavioural systems, creating a multi-dimensional relational framework that can be created anew for each individual case" (2011, p. i). An integrative approach is defined as having four distinct characteristics: 1) the viewpoint of the therapist is "holistic" seeing the individuals and groups that we work with as an integrated whole with interrelated experiences of body, mind, physiology and psychology, affective and cognitive, and physically and spiritually; 2) the integration of theories and concepts and/or techniques from different psychological and psychotherapeutic approaches; 3) the personal and professional integration of the practitioner so as to maintain an authentic, responsive, and creative contact with self and others; and 4) the integration of research and practice so that research informs practice and reflective evaluation of practice informs research.

Within the arts therapy literature in Britain, the work by Searle and Streng (2001) uses an overarching psychoanalytic theoretical frame to present a coherent paradigm for integration. This perspective grounds the work within a familiar conceptual framework that has developed within each of the creative arts therapies professions in Britain. A definition given by Searle and Streng describes how: "Integrative psychotherapy attempts to find pathways between emotions, desires, intellectual understanding, images, perceptions, and the body" (2001; p. 9). They develop themes of an interconnection between the body, the imagination, the intellect, and emotional internal experiences that the client in therapy brings to the work.

Theories that can be used to support understanding of the integration of the arts in psychotherapy are described in Chapter 3, drawing on commonalities and overlaps between the different arts therapies' theoretical ideas and applications. The relational model that provides a framework for integration at IATE is described in Chapter 4, with links made to examples of the use of the arts and how this might emerge, support, or deepen engagement with each layer of the relationship. These two chapters combined aim to provide a theoretical underpinning for safe, graduated, and explorative psychotherapy and contain the principal elements used when integrating the arts and the psychotherapy relationship.

Using all of the arts

The facilitation of creativity through a connection with various arts media provides the foundation of integrative arts psychotherapy. The creative medium used, whether through the visual arts, music, drama, or dance/movement, offers four essential therapeutic processes beyond those of a conventional verbal psychotherapy format, by providing: a) a conceptual space in which the creative arts extend a reflective narrative; b) a symbolic-creative space through which feeling is given form; c) an embodied experience of self through the sensory processes of creativity; and d) a material space through producing tangible art objects or digital recordings of the creative art process that provide a reflective container of the therapeutic journey.

The principle of an integrative therapy is based on the interplay and overlaps between the different creative and expressive art forms. Rather than viewing each art modality as separate with its unique distinct properties, an integration of the arts allows an authentic movement between different modes of expression in a client-led and collaborative exploration of creative potential.

In the integrative arts psychotherapy training at IATE, a range of art forms are integrated in practice – with the visual arts used as a shared language, in which all students have to demonstrate their proficiency. The seven art forms used are as follows: 1) the visual arts; 2) sculpture/clay; 3) bodywork/movement; 4) sand play; 5) drama/ puppetry; 6) poetry; and 7) music. The use of the visual arts can include two-dimensional imagery, mark-making, visual media, visualisation (including visual metaphors), collage, fabric, digital imagery, video, animation, and photography. Work with sculpture and clay could include three-dimensional imagery, modelling, clay work, carving or sculpting, natural object use, art making with natural materials, and earth art. The movement basis of the visual arts offers the potential to draw attention to the visual narratives and energetic quality of the artwork or shift attention to the expressive movement and dance that went into its creation. The combination of visual imagery and kinaesthetic movement produces verbal and non-verbal narratives as well as healing momentum that may generate the formation of a complementary or contrasting art form. The visual art form may lead to a movement sculpt, a dance, or a poetic response.

Bodywork, dance, and movement provide an opportunity to explore the relational "contact" between the therapist and the client through the kinaesthetic tension; this is experienced within a safe and experimental movement or dance. It is also possible to work with what the body is already communicating symbolically, whether through posture, gesture, and gait or through illness and injury. Movement is integral to the very process of change. The bodies of both the client and the therapist are highly attuned, sensory receptors of non-verbal, subjective, and creative phenomena which are sensed, felt, and experienced within the potential space held by the triangular relationship.

The use of sand play includes working with small world figures within the framed space of the sandtray in which landscapes, settings, and backdrops can be created and characters introduced. It is worth noting that the sand itself can provide a visual or sculptural medium, which can be soothing to touch and to move into shapes or forms within the containing space of the tray. The enactment of a dramatic story can be animated through the objects, characters, and animals used in the "theatre of the sandtray". Once feelings are organised and externalised in sand play, they can be contemplated from a distance and then assimilated. The images and dramatic storylines that were animated in the sandtray can lead to visual art making or written narrative and journaling.

The dramatic arts include the use of materials and visual arts media to create settings and props, puppets, shadow puppets, sound and rhythm, masks and character props. Storytelling and writing, the use of the body, the voice, and the arts are used to animate and enact the therapeutic narrative, storyline, or central metaphor. The use of dramatic and embodied metaphor can generate a visual or symbolic form that is developed further using the visual arts, and equally, a visual metaphor can be transposed from paper to movement as when facilitating the bodily enactment of an important metaphor as it is experienced in the body.

The use of poetry in therapy can emerge in response to another art form, a movement, or an image, as the poetic use of language can hold and reflect paradox, uncertainty, and ambiguity in word form. Poetry can consolidate creative presence through the playful association of words. Literal words may misrepresent, underplay, hide rather than reveal, and frequently offer only approximations to any recalled experience, while poetry, as a multi-sensorial form, may amplify and express the full, embodied experience.

Music and sound improvisation resonate and reflect the vital forms of one's felt life: the rises and falls, surges and floods, the tensions and intensities, changes in tempo, the dissonances, harmonies, and resolutions. We know these forms intimately in our emotional experiencing. Music, rhythm, and sound can convey the full qualitative and energetic aspects of an important relationship, atmosphere, crucial event, or ongoing situation. Sound is always present in the therapy relationship and can be amplified at times when it takes a step into the foreground of the work. Sound improvisation is often used to interact and interrelate with a call and response expression in both individual and groupwork contexts.

While not listed as an art form at IATE, play is seen to underpin all creativity and is a fundamental requisite within all psychotherapeutic work with all age groups and across all therapy settings. Being able to play with thoughts, ideas, and utilise the deep resource of the imagination is essential to an effective therapeutic process. Playfulness within the shared dialogue of therapy is given greater access when we establish a trusting and accepting environment in which the creative presence of the client is invited, encouraged, and responded to with curiosity. An integrative approach when using all of the arts also requires a playful, imaginative engagement of the therapist by using improvisation and spontaneity within the creative response towards the creative presence of others.

The creative arts therapies all share the significance of "embodied process". This process is described in different ways depending on the art form and theoretical perspectives used. Jones (2007) uses the term the "dramatic body" which communicates through "embodied metaphor and gesture" (Jones, 2007), Odell-Miller (2001) describes the interaction and improvisational basis of musical narratives that resonate with the body of both the therapist and the client, and art therapists work with artworks and "embodied images" that express the inner life of the client (Schaverien, 1992). What these different creative expressions of embodied experience show us is that there is a point in therapy when the internal experience of the client and the external expression through the arts resonate. This may be experienced viscerally in the body of the client and/or therapist, in a sonic frequency between the therapist and the client, or as a sense of harmony as in a pictorial or musical composition. When a resonance is present, there is usually a deeply felt expression, and both the therapist and the client experience a congruent alignment through the senses, sensations, and affects produced by an internal response within the body. The embodied experiences are held, expressed, and externalised through the different art forms. The body not only absorbs and responds to creative acts but also provides the movement and energy that underpins all the creative forms of expression. The body generates creative expression and contains the spirit, complexity, and nature of the client in therapy.

Creative integration in practice

The chapters that follow in Part III, Part IV, and Part V are all written by IATE staff and graduates. They share a series of clinical examples that describe this approach to integration in clinical thinking and the use of the arts in therapy. As each chapter unfolds, one by one, the reader will be able to begin to experience how the structural framework and integrative arts approach can enable and support therapeutic work.

In Part III, work with individuals is explored across a range of different clinical settings. An approach to using the arts and the body to assist discovery and self-awareness is explored in Chapter 5. This shows how working somatically with the arts can support the process of growth within the co-created relational field between the therapist and the client and how verbal and non-verbal communication, metaphor, emerging images, and the interchange between embodiment and externalisation enable insight offering the potential for change. Then in Chapter 6, a way to work collaboratively with clients to facilitate a movement of creative energy that is initiated, developed, and completed through the "creative cycle" is described. This work is taken from private practice with adults and uses the body, the visual arts, and metaphor within the person-to-person relationship and from a "dialogic" stance.

The therapeutic use of voice and embodied sound as a journey of integration of the self focusing especially on work with trauma survivors is explored in Chapter 7. It demonstrates how to work safely and collaboratively with the younger, wounded parts of the self, silenced by childhood trauma, supporting the client to fully own and integrate that traumatised child part into their adult being, fostering it back into the family of self. In Chapter 8, the author sets out how integrative arts psychotherapy has enabled her to work in partnership with clients who experience anxiety, depression, and suicidal ideation, providing a model for robust and rigorous clinical thinking and practice. The chapter demonstrates that a trauma-informed way of using the arts does not need to be reductive but can instead allow space for what may have remained hidden to come to light in a safe, contained, and timely way.

While the pandemic has caused many challenges for art therapists and clients, it has also inspired new ways of working and encouraged art therapists to take a flexible, creative approach when thinking about how they could work and the boundaries needed for this to be safe. In Chapter 9, the author explores working with clients online and explains how this can offer new opportunities for art therapy practice – from the initial assessment of a client's suitability for remote therapy, through contracting and documentation, and into risk assessment. She finds that digitally mediated therapy can amplify themes of presence/absence, connection/disconnection, openness/concealment, and flow/interruption. These can form part of the challenge – and the rewards – of practicing integrative arts psychotherapy online.

In Part IV, the authors go on to explore the use of this creative integrative approach when working with different groups. In Chapter 10, the personal development groups that form part of integrative arts psychotherapy training are considered. These are seen to offer a unique opportunity to develop how creative arts therapists understand issues of identity, gender, race, power, privilege, ableism, and sexuality. The author contends that it is imperative that creative arts therapists examine all aspects of their identity in therapy, and that the personal development group within therapy training is a key place where these issues can be addressed. This chapter explores some of the change processes that can take place in these group settings to address issues arising from intersectional identities and the power relations that are prevalent throughout society.

A storytelling and multi-modal arts psychotherapy group, created by collaborative dual working between an integrative arts psychotherapist and a drama psychotherapist on an older adult mental health inpatient ward, is explored in Chapter 11. The different art modalities weave together within an integrative theoretical framework, underpinned by trauma-informed practice offering choice, agency, community, and resources. The concept of liminality and rites of passage is explored in the context of working within an inpatient setting. Complex trauma, together with the many bereavements and losses faced by this age group, is considered in creating a safe therapeutic space where personal stories can find expression through graded engagement with the arts. Critical thinking is given to the importance of sharing diverse narratives within the group and the containment of intense affect through the expression of untold stories layered in multiple art forms.

In Chapter 12, a structured fixed-term group is described that draws upon advances in dual diagnosis treatment, within a residential rehab setting. The RAFT integrative arts programme moves away from the 12-step disease model of treatment, widely associated with traditional rehab programmes, focusing instead on the so-called "self-medication" hypothesis. This assumption conceptualises addiction as developing from an individual's reliance on a drug/substance to alleviate or change a range of painful affect states.

Reflections on an integrative approach and innovations in practice

The focus of Part V is reflective practice and integrating the voice of the client and the creative experiences of the therapist when evaluating practice or constructing a research design. In Chapter 14, a three-way dialogue between a service user and two integrative arts psychotherapists enables a shared reflection on therapy, collaboration, co-design, and co-production. The discussion offers a contained, creative, and reflective space to explore therapeutic practice, starting from the point of view of someone with lived experience as a service user, artist, and arts in health practitioner. The exchange aims to bring to the fore some choice points in the ways that the therapeutic relationship and using the arts as a means of communication and a support for recovery are engaged within therapy sessions and show how working together in this way can empower both the service user and the therapist.

The importance of incorporating research into practice as the way in which a new profession generates evidence, develops research methodologies, and adapts practice as new and innovative approaches emerge from clinical experiences is explained in Chapter 15. The relational focus of researching therapy considers the therapist's subjective experiences as being inextricably linked to the implicit and explicit experiences of the client in the therapy relationship. These experiences are seen as a reciprocal exchange of energy, affect, imagery, and imaginative responses that occur in the body and imagination of the therapist and are admissible as evidence and research data.

And finally, in Chapter 16, the author explains that therapists are by nature interested in stories, showing how through the pain and struggle of their own lives, they come to understand and trust the value of the stories they hear from their clients (whether revealed through words, actions, or the arts). The chapter demonstrates that formal, qualitative research is not so different from what we do as therapists within the confines of the therapy room – collaborative, working with participants in their search for the truth and meaning of personal experience.

Facilitation and improvisation

When we make art, we are in movement, and we are in feeling. We may dance as we draw, paint with rhythm, or feel a dramatic embodiment through the physicality of touching media and creating form. The elaboration of the spoken word through a visual exploration of texture and colour, or the use of objects and poetry whilst describing a personal narrative, can give shape to feeling and experience whilst amplifying their meaning through movement and dramatic expression. These subtle and intertwined visual and verbal narratives take shape and emerge through the arts in an integrative arts psychotherapy session. The questions that arise when we extend the range of potential art forms are related to the facilitation from one arts media to another.

The facilitation of a particular arts response will depend on many factors such as theoretical orientation, therapeutic methods used, choice of technique or the preferred art media, and range of materials available in the studio. The movement from talking to drawing or painting will be familiar for many art therapists. Introducing the option to physically move around the studio, an invitation to work on the wall or floor, may also be a common choice and is always a collaborative decision that is client-led. However, how would decisions to introduce modelling clay, sandtray, or natural materials be navigated? And how might one frame the suggestion of working with the voice, musical rhythm, song, or poetry? Transitioning from dramatic enrolment to claywork or from painting into body movement requires an attuned prompt, or an impromptu suggestion, sometimes client-led, at other times practitioner-led, and always as a collaborative intentional agreement. The following chapters will explore these epistemological questions and develop a multi-modal theoretical frame that underpins art-based transitions in an integrative arts psychotherapy practice.

References

Gilbert, M. & Orlans, V. (2011) *Integrative therapy: 100 key points and techniques.* Routledge.

Jones, P. (2007) *Drama as therapy: Theory, practice and research* (second edition). Routledge.

Odell-Miller, H. (2001) Music therapy and its relationship to psychoanalysis. In Searle, Y. and Streng, I. (eds.) *Where analysis meets the arts: The integration of the arts therapies with psychoanalytic theory* (pp. 127–152). Karnac Books Ltd.

Schaverien, J. (1992) *The revealing image: Analytical art psychotherapy in theory and practice*. Jessica Kingsley Publishers.

Searle, Y. & Streng, I. (eds.) (2001) *Where analysis meets the arts: The integration of the arts therapies with psychoanalytic theory*. Karnac Books Ltd.

Waller, D. (1991) *Becoming a profession: The history of art therapy in Britain 1940–1982.* Routledge.

Part I

Integrating the arts in psychotherapy

Development of an integrative approach in the UK

Chapter 1

History and development of integrative arts psychotherapy in Britain

Claire Louise Vaculik, Margot Sunderland, and Graeme Blench

Introduction

The creative therapeutic practices and approach to living that we teach at the Institute for Arts in Therapy and Education (IATE) are based upon experience and insights gained over the past 30 years, informed by an ongoing journey of exploration and discovery. All of our work at IATE has been and continues to be guided by the vision of our founders – Dr Margot Sunderland, Dr Ken Pickering, and Dr Stephen Little.

Margot, Ken, and Stephen passionately believed a healthier society to be one in which the creative working-through of emotional pain, within a safe and supportive arena, is not merely the property of a few psychologically minded people or restricted to the confines of the art gallery or theatre (IATE, 2021). They believed that it should be possible for many more people to process their feelings well, rather than simply managing them via "neurotic" or destructive means. And in setting up IATE, they aimed to explore the therapeutic application of the arts and the creative imagination for a more fulfilling life, rather than purely for remedial use or simply for addressing a particular problem (IATE, 2021). The passion and commitment to this vision have drawn in and inspired so many others – the hundreds of staff members and visiting lecturers, who chose to bring their own skills and expertise to IATE to enrich and further develop this exciting work; a wide range of organisations that have worked in partnership with us; and also, over 3,000 students who have come to study and journey with us from all across the UK and abroad.

The courses and workshops offered at IATE have changed and developed over the years, with our current portfolio providing a range of short courses and accredited vocational degree programmes that combine cutting-edge research, experiential learning, and creativity with the arts. All of our child counselling, psychotherapy, and arts psychotherapy trainings continue to provide our students with the skills to make a real difference in other people's lives and to develop a truly fulfilling career (IATE, 2020). We work hard to stay at the forefront of a changing and developing field, as we want to support our students and graduates to be able to identify and use the most appropriate and effective practice in

DOI: 10.4324/9781003155676-3

all that they do. The majority of our tutors and visiting lecturers are practising clinicians and many teach internationally. On the Integrative Arts Psychotherapy course specifically, we also draw upon the experiences and expertise of service users, art therapists with dual experience, arts in health practitioners, researchers, and a wide range of other professionals. This helps us to ensure that our graduates always put service users at the heart of all that they do, empowering these unique individuals to work collaboratively within the therapeutic relationship across the therapeutic journey. It also supports students' growing understanding of the complexity and multidisciplinary nature of contemporary art therapy and psychotherapy practice and ensures that they are able to communicate effectively with other professionals working in a range of different contexts and a variety of roles (IATE, 2020).

Our students have told us that the process of undertaking their training at the Institute has deeply enriched and enhanced not only their working life but also their personal relationships and their own creative practice too. This feedback is so important to us. It demonstrates that in this shared and challenging creative work, we are living out our values and continuing to bring our founders' vision to life.

Our shared history

Much like that of a family, or a small community, the story of our work at IATE and how this developed has many layers to it. Of necessity, it also contains within it different perspectives. Our story has been shaped not only by passionate individuals who had the courage to venture into new terrain but also by differences of opinion and even disagreement – sometimes within IATE and at other times, with individuals and other organisations within the wider professional landscape that we occupy. In recording her seminal history of art therapy as a profession, Waller (1991) chose to use Bucher and Strauss' process model of professions as this allowed her to better understand diversity and the conflicts of interests that can give rise to missions within a profession, seen in terms of "segments, missions, and evolution, and in relationship to the political and economic fluctuations of a given society" (Waller, 1991, xiv). She saw this model as useful because it is able to contain the differences in opinion and conflict that arise within any profession and to view these in a positive light, as a possible source of growth or development for that profession. In this way, we suppose that our story could be seen as one such "mission", which forms an integral part of the wider history of psychotherapy and of art therapy in the UK.

Our work and the integrative approach that we have developed at IATE have been viewed by colleagues from other organisations and other professions in many different ways over the years. Some have been surprised and delighted by our approach, using this to expand their own range as a clinician or deciding to work with us in some way. Others have seen our work as being "different" and even questioned the validity of our practice, or our right to occupy certain forums.

Our commitment to our clients and to listening to their lived experience of what helps and what supports them has sustained us through some of the more challenging times. We know that our practice is informed by a close attention to what they tell us works for them, by a commitment to rigour, by relevant best practice guidelines, and by emerging research findings. And that it is enlivened by our creativity, playfulness, curiosity, and determination to live out our values in the support of others.

It is possible that this book about our work may inspire debate within the profession and we welcome that. Hogan (2009, pp. 29–30) developed a useful tool to reflect on the diversity of art therapy practice in the UK, which she called the art therapy continuum. She noted that some art therapists had reported to her that they had "found it helpful in helping them think about where they stand" (Hogan, 2009, p. 30). We hope that this chapter and this book might be helpful in a similar manner.

We believe that it is vital that art therapists remain at the forefront of psychotherapy practice and continue to offer the most appropriate and effective interventions, supporting their clients to gain self-awareness, to grow, and to change – informed by the latest research, by developing best practice from across the globe, and by their own lived experience of being courageous, creative, and engaged human beings.

We want to share our way of working with you so that you can see the vision that inspires us, engage with our story, and understand integrative arts psychotherapy practice. We are passionate about our clients, about IATE, and about this profession. We hope that this process of sharing, comparison, and critical engagement with our model will inspire and challenge you in equal measure. Perhaps, it will enable you to locate where you "stand" and to reflect anew on your own ways of working, nourishing you in your ongoing development as a clinician. It might help to identify different choice points in practice, or perhaps inspire you to see new creative possibilities that might enrich and develop your own work with service users. Whatever the impact, we hope that learning about our work will mean that you start to build a relationship with us and that this rich contact can, in turn, inform, challenge, shape, and influence our own IAP practice in the future.

Early days: setting up the Institute for Arts in Therapy and Education

The history of IATE and the integrative arts psychotherapy approach that developed there has arisen from a rich ground of friendships, partnerships, and chance encounters, underpinned by an abiding passion for helping others, a belief in the power of the arts to support transformation and change, and a commitment to rigorous, creative exploration.

In 1986, Margot Sunderland and Ken Pickering were working together as colleagues in Canterbury. Margot had trained originally in dance and was lecturing on a Performing Arts Degree course at Nonington College, awarded by the

University of Kent. This is where she met Ken, a Principal Lecturer in Drama and Performance at the University of Kent, who had a similar passion for creativity.

Over time Margot found that she became increasingly interested in the therapeutic potential of the arts, starting a gestalt psychotherapy course at Metanoia Psychotherapy Training Institute – a humanistic psychotherapy and counselling school (Watt, 2019). She was working therapeutically with adolescents in residential units, using sand play therapy, art, movement, and puppets. Dr Stephen Little, a child and adolescent psychiatrist and psychoanalytic psychotherapist, had been providing clinical supervision for Margot and Graeme Blench, a music therapist working in the adolescent units with her. Dr Little found the multi-arts approach that they were using with young people very interesting and effective, and in conversation with Margot and Ken, he sparked the plan to develop their shared interests and set up a new project together.

In a discussion that took place at Dr Little's oast house in Kent, they reflected on what had been helpful and effective in supporting young people from these very challenging backgrounds. Dr Little shared his view that the arts were the way forward and that a multi-arts approach – using the visual arts, sculpture, bodywork and movement, sand play, drama and puppetry, poetry, and music – seemed to have been of most benefit to enable self-expression, self-exploration, and healing. They knew that offering only one art form would not have served the teenagers well, as some of the teenagers chose to work with music as their main therapeutic tool, some sand play, and others chose art or clay.

Margot and Ken agreed and they decided to develop a series of different workshops in Canterbury to share some of their experiences of using all of the arts in this way with others. The work developed organically, starting with a one-day series of workshops at Kent University. This quickly sold out, with over 200 attendees. People seemed to recognise the value of the work right away and wanted to learn more. After this initial success, Margot and Ken went on to develop the first course and hired a small, rather draughty, church hall in Canterbury to run the teaching days. They called this course the Certificate in Therapeutic Arts. The first cohort in September 1986 had eight people enrolled, and the training was later validated by the London College of Dance and Drama. Dr Little was involved with this work for the first year or so.

Not everyone was as pleased about these developments, with some music therapists, art therapists, and drama therapists writing to the College's Principal to object to a multi-arts course being run there. The work continued to develop and grow though and, over time, Margot and Ken started to approach other professionals to join them in teaching the course.

In early 1987, Margot approached a music therapist to offer some teaching on the course about the therapeutic use of music. She refused, as the students were not trained musicians. Margot then asked Graeme Blench, her colleague in the adolescent unit, if he would consider providing some workshops. Having seen the benefits that a multi-arts approach had brought for the young people where they worked together, Graeme agreed.

After running the certificate course in Canterbury, Margot and Ken had a clearer sense of what they wanted to achieve over the longer term. They decided that they would start an organisation, which would be called the Institute for Arts in Therapy and Education, with a focus on both therapy and education. This was particularly important to Ken, as he hoped that the work could have a wider relevance than just in the consulting room.

Margot and Ken developed a post-graduate course, with the support of Professor Malcolm Ross – Honorary Research Fellow at the University of Exeter. He had run the first national curriculum research project on the arts in schools, based at Dartington College of Arts. He was the author of books that had greatly influenced Margot – *The Arts and Personal Growth* (1980) and *The Aesthetic Impulse* (1984). Malcolm was the founding Chair of the National Association for the Arts in Education and was appointed Reader in Arts Education at Exeter in 1987.

The MEd degree in Therapy and Education was validated by the University of Exeter. Both Margot and Ken were thrilled that University had taken on the course, particularly after some of the more hostile reactions that they'd had to manage. The training was run by IATE in London. As there wasn't a fixed building or space yet, they used different venues in London, hiring suitable rooms for each of the training days. Sadly after about four years, the University of Exeter's validation policy changed; they no longer wanted external partnerships, such as the one with IATE.

In 1989, Margot and Ken moved their work to Regents College London, which provided a much appreciated "home" for several years and a good venue for teaching. The staff team was small, with lectures and workshops provided by Margot, Graeme, Sue Rennie (a music therapist), and Francesca Raphael (an art therapist and now, psychoanalyst). Margot remembers well the excitement of being allocated a large walk-in storeroom for equipment at Regents, after moving between hired spaces for so long. She explained: "This meant that instead of bringing all of the art materials and equipment in every time, they were there on the premises! It was like, we have a store room, wow! We've made it!" The team was able to use the surrounding gardens too, so the training was developed to include workshops outdoors in Regents Park.

But, there were some practical challenges to be overcome in delivering the course. Few other programmes at Regents College offered expressive, creative workshops, and the buildings weren't really designed for this sort of work. So after a few happy years there, staff began to notice some tensions with other trainings that worked in adjoining rooms. After a particularly exuberant and impactful drumming workshop, there were a number of complaints. Margot realised that the work was growing and developing and that in order to realise its potential fully, they would need to find separate, permanent premises for IATE. She asked a colleague, Simon Harrison, to look into suitable buildings. In 1992, he found an old dilapidated printing factory in Islington, just off Essex Road.

This empty shell of a building was to become the London ArtHouse, where IATE is still located today. At the start, Simon showed her just one floor (with space for three large training rooms and an office). Margot stood outside the building that first day and said: "We're going to have all of it you know!"

The organisation was very small, and the founders took part in all of the staff meetings, talking about the work and about how best to support students to grow and develop. Early tutors, like Tsafi Lederman, described it as being "like a small family". Tsafi had first come to know the building when she hired a space to run a group for osteopaths. At that time, she was a UKCP psychotherapist and a trainer for body psychotherapy. While running her groups, she noticed all of the other art materials and was drawn to the IATE way of working. She decided to do the training, using APL to join the third year, and after completing this started to teach on the course.

At that time, there was still a printing factory in one part of the building. As space became available though, it was taken on, refurbished and decorated – soon Margot's dream had become reality. As the space expanded, the work at IATE was able to grow and grow too, with larger conferences being arranged.

Developing and changing in response to student feedback, the focus of the work at IATE was becoming more clinical. IATE decided to apply to join the United Kingdom Standing Conference for Psychotherapy in 1992. This body had been set up following the Foster Report (1971) and the Sieghart Report (1978) recommendations for the regulation of the psychotherapy field; it later became the United Kingdom Council for Psychotherapy (Feltham, 2013, p. 9). A larger child psychotherapy training organisation tried to stop IATE from joining, and Margot remembers feeling thrilled when their application was finally approved. The first UKCP accredited psychotherapy course at IATE, run at the Islington premises, had five students on it.

Developing an approach using all of the arts

In the early days, the founders' focus was on bringing the richness of all of the seven art forms together, as this was what seemed to most benefit clients. They could see the healing that came from engaging creatively and playfully with these different art materials and then, from this base, with life more broadly. Each art form – visual arts, sculpture, bodywork and movement, sand play, drama and puppetry, poetry, and music – offered different, exciting possibilities for therapeutic work. Using them together, with a spirit of playful exploration, seemed to deepen and develop the work even further. All seven art forms used in the training were engaged fully from the start, but the thinking about how or when to move from one art form to the next to develop integration in the approach was still developing.

To help them to understand what seemed to be happening in the arts and in the relationship that led to and supported growth and change, Margot and Ken used a wide range of theories of creativity, psychotherapeutic theory, and ideas from philosophy. Over time, the emphasis on psychoanalytic thinking grew. Margot was passionate about these ideas, as they had helped her so much in her own development – she was in psychoanalysis five times a week for many years and regularly attended lectures at the Institute for Psychoanalysis. She was also passionate about gestalt theory and saw how this informed her use of the arts in sessions with clients. In addition, John Hood Williams was providing private teaching for her on sand play therapy; John had succeeded Margaret Lowenfeld as Director of the Institute for Child Psychology, the first child psychotherapy course in the UK. Lowenfeld was also the founder of sand play therapy. All of these loves influenced and informed the integrative arts psychotherapy approach, as it was being developed. Later transactional analysis was included in the curriculum too, as these ideas seemed to be really helpful for students and could also be used as a form of psycho-education in sessions to support clients to understand and articulate their own experiences.

When new staff members joined the team, they brought different skills and knowledge to the trainings and as people changed, some of the priorities changed; at times, there was discussion about which approach was more dominant. Staff today still have these rich and interesting conversations in the staff room, which spur us on to develop our practice further.

This passion for drawing on both psychodynamic and humanistic theory informed the work, enabling practitioners to work appropriately with relationship patterns developed in early life that persist in the present while holding in mind human potential and the possibility of transformation and change. That said, it was evident that taking an eclectic approach using such different theories was sometimes confusing for clients and a lack of overall integration in the thinking about the work also made it more difficult to manage risk and to pace and grade interventions in sessions. Margot realised that they needed to find a suitable framework for integration, which could underpin thinking and practice.

A framework for integration

Influenced by her own training at Metanoia and some of the discussions that had taken place there, Margot approached Petruska Clarkson, who had been inspired by Gelso and Carter's (1985) exposition of the working alliance, person-to-person relationship, transference relationship, and transpersonal relationship. Petruska used this and reflections on her own practice to expand their work to consider a multiplicity of psychotherapeutic relationships (Clarkson, 1989, 1991):

1   The working alliance
2   The person-to-person relationship
3   The reparative/developmentally-needed relationship
4   The transference/counter-transference relationship
5   The transpersonal relationship.

Petruska was interested in a multi-arts approach and agreed to come and teach this framework to students at IATE, in order to support and develop the growing theoretical integration underpinning their practice.

Later influences

At this time, Margot was still doing a lot of the teaching at IATE and inspired students with her passion and energy. She was supported in this by Graeme, who provided music therapy workshops and lectures on psychoanalytic theory, transactional analysis, and philosophy. His keen intellectual rigour, insight, humour, and quirky perspectives on IAP practice were, and continue to be, much appreciated by students and by staff.

Margot and Graeme were joined by a small group of psychotherapists, some early graduates of IATE and others from Metanoia – these included two of the co-founders (Sue Fish and Maria Gilbert) and other trainers (like Charlotte Sills and Jenny Mackewn). Margot remembers Maria Gilbert's support in clinical supervision as being invaluable for the development of IATE. Maria's varied experience meant they could use their time to explore clinical work and also to reflect on developing and running psychotherapy trainings and managing complex organisational dynamics.

Brett Kahr, a psychoanalytical psychotherapist, also trained at IATE in the early years. Years later, after a series of rich discussions about the work that was being done at IATE and how this supported clients, he suggested introducing Margot to a number of other like-minded psychoanalytic psychotherapists. Together they mapped out some possible connections – on the tablecloth in a restaurant in Hampstead! This led to a period of exchange and cross-fertilisation.

Margot also started looking abroad for work that seemed to resonate with what IATE staff, graduates, and students were finding best served their clients. She invited both UK and international speakers to come to IATE to provide lectures and speak at conferences at the London Arthouse. These days were often attended by several hundred people, including IATE students, colleagues, and members of the public. Some of the early speakers included, amongst many others, Prof Leslie Greenberg, Lolita Sapriel, Joseph Zinker, Shaun McNiff, and Prof Colwyn Trevarthen. Margot was particularly excited when Shaun McNiff agreed to come over to London. She'd read his book, "Art as Medicine", when it was published in 1993 and notes: "I immediately recognised a similar approach. It was like, that's what we think! It's about using all the arts".

After reading up about some of the research findings and developments in the field of neuroscience and looking at links with trauma, Margot decided that this was an important addition to the literature that would impact therapeutic practice. In 1998, she made contact with Jaak Panksepp and started to focus on affective neuroscience. She had private tutorials with Panksepp for many years, and he came and spoke at the Institute several times. Over the years that followed, she also invited Dr Alan Schore, Prof Bessel van der Kolk, Dr Bruce Perry, Dr Allan Schore, Dr Stephen Porges, Dr Martin Teicher, and Prof Antonio Damasio to present. Students gained immeasurably from this direct contact with some of the foremost thinkers in the field at the time.

Developing a separate child psychotherapy training

Although initially working with children, young people, and adults, the team started to notice some important differences in working with children. They also noted the increase in demand for specific child-focused courses.

At that time, there was one MA programme at IATE, which was validated by London Metropolitan University, leading to UKPC registration through HIPC. In 1999, the team started to develop an additional module that could be added on to the integrative arts psychotherapy training. This would enable graduates to be well prepared for working with children, as the team believed strongly that more specialist skills and knowledge were needed to practice child psychotherapy.

This child module was later developed into the MA in Integrative Child Psychotherapy, led by Sue Fish until her death (BGJ, 2001). Sue was really the pioneer of humanistic child psychotherapy. After her death, the child course was run Sue Harris, later by Pat Bryant (who also came to IATE from Metanoia), until being taken over in 2010 by an IATE graduate, Roz Read.

IATE wanted to accredit the child course with the UKCP so that it could lead to registration as a child psychotherapist. The Association of Child Psychotherapy (ACP), which was a member organisation of UKCP at the time, did not support this. IATE was the first organisation, outside the Anna Freud Centre and the Tavistock, able to award qualifications for child psychotherapy. The ACP later left UKCP and set up a separate register for child and adolescent psychotherapists. A number of graduates who'd completed the child module were then "grandparented" onto the UKCP register as child psychotherapists.

As the trainings grew and developed, more and more graduates gained experience in integrative arts psychotherapy and many came back to teach at IATE. Jocelyn James (later Samuels, now Quennell), a dramatherapist and IAP graduate, became the programme director of the MA in Integrative Arts Psychotherapy. She was passionate about Jungian theory and introduced more teaching on Jung into the curriculum. The organisation's work became more complex too and Sherla Richardson joined IATE, bringing much-valued skills as an experienced business manager. Margot continued in her role as Principal, Graeme joined the Senior Management Team, and Ken served on the IATE Academic Board.

The HCPC and the introduction of the protected title: art therapist/arts psychotherapist

In 2002, the Health Professions Council was set up under the National Health Service Reform and Health Care Professions Act, to replace the Council for Professions Supplementary to Medicine (CPSM). A group of allied health professions joined the statutory register and these professional titles were protected by law. From the time that art therapist/arts psychotherapist became a protected title,

IATE began to receive complaints about graduates using their UKCP-registration descriptor, integrative arts psychotherapist.

Margot was the Principal at this time, but she later stepped down and the role was taken up by the adult training course leader, Jocelyn Samuels. As the number of challenges increased, IATE contacted the HPC and shared the history of their UKCP registration and their designated descriptor. After some discussion with Prof Diane Waller, who was a visitor for the HPC, it was suggested that IATE should apply to have the training approved. As a dramatherapist herself, Jocelyn could see the range of benefits that this might offer graduates.

The first application was refused. Mary Holyoake later joined IATE as Academic Registrar, and she took on the lengthy process of applying for approval a second time. The existing programme met the standards of education and training for the UKCPs Humanistic and Integrative College, so adjustments had to be made to meet the HPC SETs. The application was submitted, followed by a visit in October 2006. The HPC report (2006) from this visit notes that IATE would be required to revise the assessment design to require that at least two practical assessments are undertaken using the art therapy modality specifically – both assessments must use the visual art modality, at least one of these assessments must be in the final year of training, and no more than one may use the sand play modality. The visitors believed that this condition would ensure that future graduates would all have to demonstrate specific competency in the art therapy modality.

These changes were made, and after this, approval was granted. This meant that students enrolling in the training in the 2007/8 academic year would be able to join the HPC register when they graduated in the summer of 2010. Unfortunately, any previous graduates, or students already enrolled in the training, would not be able to apply for HPC registration. As these graduates' registration was with the UKCP, their professional descriptor would remain "integrative arts psychotherapists". This historic overlap between titles used by the statutory and voluntary registers continues to cause some confusion, right up to the present day.

Changes in course leadership

In 2007, Jocelyn Samuels left her role as Principal of IATE but continued in her role as programme leader through the following academic year. In 2008, she attended the British Association of Art Therapists (BAAT) AGM at the request of Val Huet, then CEO of BAAT. Val explained to members that Jocelyn had been invited to talk to BAAT members as the recent intake of students at IATE would be able to register with HPC when they graduated and as such, also able to join BAAT as members. The AGM report, published in the BAAT magazine "Newsbriefing" noted, "it therefore felt useful to open up a dialogue with IATE especially as past relationships had not always been cordial" (BAAT, 2009, p. 16). IATE staff from that time agree that there had been a range of challenges to overcome in building relationships with art therapists who were less familiar with the IAP approach, or who may have had some reservations about the programme becoming HPC approved.

Jocelyn Samuels later stood down as Programme Leader, which triggered a Major Change process and a visit from the HPC. It was proposed that the role be taken on by Chris Rowan, an HPC dramatherapist, working in collaboration with Lynne Gerlach. Lynne was described in the HPC report as "an IATE trained integrative arts psychotherapist" (HPC, 2007), though she is a Metanoia-trained gestalt psychotherapist. Some concerns were raised by the HPC at the time of this Major Change process, which focused on: the rationale for having two programme leaders and how this joint role would be managed in practice; how the registered programme leader, as a dramatherapist, would input into driving the art therapy profession specific knowledge, skills, and agenda throughout the programme; and the number of registered art therapists teaching on the programme (HPC, 2008). While the job share was approved by the HPC in the end, they specified that more art therapists should be recruited to teach on the programme. Art therapists were already providing some teaching on the programme, for example, Marrianne Behm, a Goldsmiths-trained art therapist, taught and continues to teach regularly on the course. She had first joined IATE in early 2007, as a placement coordinator for the child programme. Marrianne started to teach some sessions on both programmes, including lectures on the history of art therapy and object relations theory.

The Programme Leader job-share arrangement appears to have been challenging to manage, and it only lasted one academic year. Both post holders lived far away from London and from each other. They also had to manage two very different sets of standards of education and training, which were not easy to reconcile in practice. After they stepped down, it was hoped that having one person in this role, who understood both of these registers well, might make the process easier to contain and manage in practice. This seemed particularly important as the debate was raging within the UKCP about the possibility of statutory regulation through the HPC being extended to psychotherapy and counselling, with very strong views being expressed on both sides.

In 2009, IATE approached Claire Louise Leyland (now Vaculik) and asked if she would be prepared to interview for the post. She was at that time one of a small number of therapists who had both HPC registration as an art therapist (trained in a psychodynamic approach at Goldsmiths College) and UKCP registration, through the HIPC (trained as a gestalt psychotherapist at Metanoia Institute). Claire Louise was passionate about working in an integrative way, using a range of art forms to support clients' creative engagement in therapy, and adapting her practice to best suit the particular needs of the client or group. She accepted this new challenge, as it would enable her to develop these interests and share ideas with others. She started in her post as Programme Director in the 2009/10 academic year and has worked closely with Margot Sunderland and Graeme Blench since this time, aiming to ensure that the ethos of the organisation and the founders' aims continued to be embedded in any developments of the programme.

At this time, the course was still using Clarkson's (1989) five-relationship framework to support the integration of a range of theoretical approaches and all seven art forms – art, sculpture/clay, bodywork/movement, sand play, drama/ puppetry, poetry, and music. After reviewing all of the final year students' assessments, Claire Louise asked to introduce some additional content to the curriculum. She aimed to highlight the importance of undertaking rigorous assessments, understanding and managing risk, and using an evidence-based approach to inform clinical work. As an active member of her professional body, then recently co-opted on BAAT Council, Claire Louise also wanted to start to help the IATE graduates who would now be joining the art therapy profession to better understand the professional landscape in which they would be working. She believed strongly that art therapists really needed to be creative and entrepreneurial in all of their practice, not just in therapy. As a project manager with experience in writing bids, she wanted to equip IATE graduates to develop the kind of new and inspiring projects that would meet the particular needs of their communities across the UK.

She also started to invite more art therapy colleagues (like Fran la Nave, Gary Nash, Val Huet, and Joan Woddis) to come and teach at IATE. Many had previously worked with or supervised students and graduates, which had piqued their interest in the integrative approach.

Deepening and developing the IAP approach

From 2011, Claire Louise introduced Gilbert and Orlans' (2010) six-relationship framework to the programme, as this framework developed Clarkson's work to support a stronger focus on cultural awareness and thinking about the impact of difference on the therapeutic relationship. Dr Vanja Orlans taught and continues to teach this framework to incoming IAP students each year.

In 2013, Ken left the Academic Board. It was a time of change, and the partnership with London Met ended too. The programme was re-written and then validated by the University of East London. Aiming to encourage more diversity in the student body and to support people on their paths through the training journey, each year of training was structured as a separate module. This meant that students who completed the foundation, the first year of the MA, and 100 hours of supervised placement could exit their credits and take these to register with the BACP as a counsellor. Some students do choose to do this each year. Then after a few years, when they are able to do so, many return to IATE to complete their MA and register with the Health and Care Professions Council (the HPC was renamed, HCPC in 2012). Later, once they've gained 450 hours of supervised clinical practice, they may also choose to register with the UKCP. Practice placements were also structured differently for the UEL course so that each student now completes a six-month placement in a community or voluntary sector organisation, a second year-long placement in a statutory sector organisation (e.g., NHS, prison) as part of a multidisciplinary team, and a third year-long placement that they set up themselves in a setting of their choice. From the second year of the MA, which is their third year in the psychotherapy training, students are also able to apply for permission to work in private practice – this is accepted practice on the UKCP psychotherapy training pathway. The range of placement experience aims to support all students to understand the differing policy frameworks and processes used in different sectors and to manage risk with care, understanding the wider mental health and social care system in which their particular practice is situated.

In 2020, Jude Smit (an IATE graduate) joined the team as Deputy Programme Director. This was timely as it really supported the team's work over lockdown, when many changes and adjustments were needed to teaching, learning, and placement practice. Online therapy training was introduced and offered to all staff and students in April 2020, run by another graduate Emma Cameron.

A new core module has been introduced for this academic year that considers the impact of social injustice on mental health. Margot developed this after noting that epidemiological studies show that mental health problems are far more prevalent in those who have encountered adverse experiences of discrimination, intolerance of difference, stigma, social exclusion, marginalisation, and/or micro-aggressions. Margot had been inspired and so impacted by the work that an IATE graduate, Anthea Benjamin, was doing for the UKCP on diversity and discrimination. Also, from her own ongoing work developing a range of trauma-informed courses, having won a Big Lottery Bid to deliver trauma-informed training to teachers in every school in Cornwall. The social injustice module aims to support students to consider social systems and all elements of communities in which people live, as these are interdependent and interact in complex ways. This encourages students to investigate and conduct research into global issues of social injustice and its impact on mental health and they also present their ideas to a forum of their peers.

Conclusion

In writing this chapter, we wanted to share our story with you so that you can see Margot, Ken, and Stephen's vision, engage with the path we have travelled, and understand contemporary integrative arts psychotherapy practice. We hope that this has been interesting, enabling you to reflect on the wider history of our profession through a different lens. Perhaps, it might have had echoes or resonances with the history and development of your approach to practice, or perhaps it might offer a different voice or a different perspective on the story that you were told when training.

Our work at IATE and on the integrative arts psychotherapy training has gone from strength to strength over the past 30 years. Our model is now well established, and our graduates work across all sectors, many setting up their own services, organisations, or holding management and senior leadership roles. The integrative nature of the training and recording of clinical sessions mean that all students have to reflect carefully on their approach and how work in therapy unfolds, from moment to moment. They must explain the thinking behind their use of the arts and the therapeutic relationship to assessors or groups of other students in a "live" discussion of the material in assessments. They are also required to identify alternative perspectives and choice points in the work. Using an integrative approach has tended to mean that our graduates not only have to question their assumptions and look at their work from a range of different perspectives, but also to be able to explain and justify their clinical thinking to others in a grounded and confident manner.

We hope that you will be able to use this time with us, reflecting on our journey, as a source of nourishment and that it provides food for thought. Perhaps this might also inspire you to reflect again upon your own journey and on your own model of practice, comparing this with the IAP approach and considering if any parts of this way of working could support you, as you continue to support clients on your ongoing journey of development as a practitioner.

References

British Association of Art Therapists (2009) "BAAT AGM 2008", *Newsbriefing: Spring 2009*, p. 16.

British Gestalt Journal (2001) "Sue Fish 1946–2001", *British Gestalt Journal*, 10(2), p. 78.

Clarkson, P. (1989) *Gestalt Counselling in Action*. London: Sage.

Clarkson, P. (1991) "Multiplicity of psychotherapeutic relationships", *British Journal of Psychotherapy*, 7(Winter, 2), pp. 148–163.

Feltham, C. (2013) "The cultural context of British psychotherapy", in Dryden, W. and Reeves, A. (eds.) *The Handbook of Individual Therapy*. 6th ed. London: Sage.

Foster, J. (December 1971) *Enquiry into the Practice and Effects of Scientology*. London: Her Majesty's Stationery Office.UK National Archive piece reference MH 153/606.

Gelso, C.J. and Carter, J.A. (1985) "The relationship in counseling and psychotherapy: Components, consequences, and theoretical antecedents", *The Counseling Psychologist*, 13(2), pp. 155–243.

Gilbert, M. and Orlans, V. (2010) *Integrative Therapy: 100 Key Points and Techniques*. London: Routledge.

Hogan, S. (2009) "The art therapy continuum: A useful tool for envisaging the diversity of practice in British art therapy", *International Journal of Art Therapy: Formerly Inscape*, 14(1), pp. 29–37.

HPC (2006) *Health Professions Council Approvals Panel 10 October 2006 – Visitors' Report and Representations*. Available at: www.hcpc-uk.org/globalassets/meetings-attachments3/approvals-committee/2006/october/approvals_panel_20061010_enclo sure05/ (Accessed: 6th September 2021).

HPC (2007) *Health Professions Council Education and Training Panel 28 March 2007 – Approval Visit Report*. Available at: www.hcpc-uk.org/globalassets/meetings-attachments3/education-and-training-committee/2007/march/education_and_training_panel_20070328_enclosure07/ (Accessed: 2nd January 2021).

HPC (2008) *Health Professions Council Education & Training Panel Monday 4 February 2008 – Major Change Report*. Available at: www.hcpc-uk.org/globalassets/meetings-attachments3/education-and-training-committee/2008/february/education_and_training_panel_20080204_enclosure09/ (Accessed: 2nd January 2021).

Institute for Arts in Therapy and Education (2020) *MA in Integrative Arts Psychotherapy: Student Handbook 2020/2021*. Available at: https://www.artspsychotherapy.org/art-therapy-/-arts-psychotherapy/masters-degree-in-integrative-arts-psychotherapy.

Institute for Arts in Therapy and Education (2021) *The Seven Art Forms for Therapeutic Conversation*. Available at: www.artspsychotherapy.org/iate-training/trainings-in-art-therapy-arts-psychotherapy-counselling-using-the-arts (Accessed: 7th September 2021).

Ross, M. (1980) *The Arts and Personal Growth: Curriculum Issues in Arts Education*. Ann Arbor, MI: University of Michigan, Pergamon Press.

Ross, M. (1984) *The Aesthetic Impulse*. Ann Arbor, MI: University of Michigan, Pergamon Press.

Sieghart, P. (1978) *Statutory Registration of Psychotherapists: A Report of a Professions Joint Working Party*. London: Mr S. G. Gray, Secretary of the Working Party, Tavistock Centre.

Waller, D. (1991) *Becoming a Profession: The History of Art Therapy in Britain 1940–1982*. London: Tavistock, Routledge.

Watt, L. (2019) *The Founders of Metanoia Institute: Remembered for Pride Jubilee – the 50th Anniversary of LGBT+ Pride*. Available at: https://metanoia.ac.uk/prospective-students/equality-and-diversity/equality-and-diversity-events/lgbtqplus-article/ (Accessed: 6th September 2021).

Chapter 2

Transformation across the art forms

Metamorphosis and motif

Marrianne Behm

Why integrative arts rather than single modalities? This chapter explores the answer to this question by following the journey of a National Health Service (NHS) arts psychotherapies service in the context of changes in healthcare and psychological therapies over the last 25 years. These changes have made the case for an integrative approach more pertinent and more possible. I have also added to this, my own personal journey as a clinician, not only as a way of explaining how my ideas developed but also because I want to tell this story from the inside as well as the outside. What emerges is the idea of a motif travelling across different art forms, moving inside and outside the body and inside and outside symbolic communication, towards coherence.

One of my earliest memories is chasing a mirage of dancing figures in the Australian outback before they disappeared. Their dancing seemed an attempt to fill the vast surrounding space. Dance, a visual image, and the movement of my chase came together at that moment as a single thing. I also felt a sense of something on the horizon that was out of reach yet was also a part of me; the figures were from my imagination and my imagination felt freed.

Coming to the UK as a young adult, I found myself in a very different landscape. The closeness of buildings and people meant there was no empty space for my imagination to fill. To cope, I began to doodle in my work breaks. I felt the need to make the images big and was able to blow them up to poster size, using machines in a nearby architectural practice. Enlarging kept the shape of the motif, but something was transformed: it felt like my body was diving inside the image. I had a sense of movement and rhythm, which I found therapeutic. This helped me adapt to my new landscape and propelled me to do an art psychotherapy training. I also continued to explore movement through Contact Improvisation and Laban.

Establishing an arts psychotherapy service

After qualifying, I began working as an art psychotherapist for an inner-city NHS Trust. Many of my outpatient clients were people with severe complex needs. The approach I had been trained in typically involved offering art materials, observing, and then verbally exploring the material. However, this rather analytical model

DOI: 10.4324/9781003155676-4

often created anxiety, defensiveness, and paranoia, for example, I vividly recall one client drawing a page of staring eyes. I realised I needed to adapt my approach.

I began to introduce breathing and movement to help ground people in their bodies before they engaged in art. This seemed to create a sense of trust and appeared to improve the ability to make sense of feeling through art making. However, this was the mid-1990s – the Institute of Arts in Therapy and Education (IATE) training was still in its infancy, and little was written about integrative arts approaches. There was also no arts therapy department, just two art therapists stretched across many services.

Over the next five years, successful pilot projects led to increased funding and the number of art therapists grew sufficiently to enable us to form an arts therapies department. This created a space for us to discuss and refine our approaches. Furthermore, whilst the department was initially exclusively staffed by art therapists, over time, drama therapists and dance movement therapists joined us and the door was open for us to integrate the different art forms.

However, we did not walk through this open door immediately. The arts therapies have a history of specialisation, possibly because it was felt that this gave them credibility compared with other specialised disciplines. In the UK, each of the arts therapies (dance movement, drama, music, and art) has its own training and professional association, and usually, students are expected to be competent in their modality (HCPC Standards of Practice). Given this context, it was not surprising that, initially, the therapists in our department tended to become quite territorial, guarding the boundaries of their practice fiercely, and despite my hopes for an integrative approach, the different arts therapies remained separate and specialised.

Nevertheless, other developments were taking place in parallel. The NHS was becoming increasingly concerned with Accident and Emergency (A&E) waiting times and the large number of frequent A&E attenders, who had medically unexplained physical symptoms (Parsonage and Fossey, 2011). Most of this cohort were perceived to have underlying mental health problems and there was a renewed interest in the mind–body connection.

Furthermore, developments in neuroscience supported the emergence of new treatments, which offered a bridge between mind and body such as mindfulness and new approaches to trauma (Rothchild, 2000; Van Der Kolk, 2014). During this period IATE, the only course in the UK at that time championing a multimodal approach to the arts therapies was also flourishing and teaching neuroscience as part of its training. In 2006, I became a course lecturer. This exposed me to a vast range of integrative arts work in action, as well as offering me a place to discuss and develop my practice.

Sandtray and projective objects

As a result of my IATE work, I introduced sandtray and projective object work (Lowenfeld, 2005) into my department. This proved a good place to start our integrative journey. The micro-world of projective objects and the sandtray is safe, contained, and bridges modalities. Furthermore, like art therapy, you can stand back from an arrangement of objects, creating perspective. Like dance movement therapy, there is a closeness to the body (objects can be touched and held). Like music therapy, dramatherapy, and dance movement therapy, there is a greater sense of the temporal. Like dramatherapy, these tools foreground a sense of role and narrative.

Whilst the use of projective objects was not novel, what was new was their use, in our NHS department, by art and dance movement psychotherapists and, as practice developed, these therapists began to be able to reach clients in new ways. For example, in an inpatient group, a client chose a shell as her projective object, representing a need to protect herself, and placed it outside a cluster of objects chosen by other group members. Normally, the art therapist facilitating the group would have worked with the representation statically. However, influenced by the ideas of movement and the body (Payne, 1992), the therapist offered the client the opportunity to move both herself and the object. Walking around the collection of objects, the client moved the shell back and forth, in a kind of dance between isolation and proximity to the other objects. After each movement, the client would stand back and observe the object arrangement. Finally, she noticed another shell in the object cluster that her shell could be close to and settled on a position. After this session, the client sat for the first time in the group circle and became less isolated on the ward.

Notably, the client not only was physically immersed in moving the object but also stood back to view it from a distance. Arguably, it is this interplay between working in a physically embodied way and being able to stand back from a static image that facilitated a change in the client. This way of thinking was new for us, which is not to say that our art therapists had ignored the body or that the dance movement therapists were unable to work with static images. It is more the case that working across modalities allowed more possibilities to do this and this was not really something we had articulated or conceptualised previously.

As I have discussed, possibly this reluctance to conceptualise the place where boundaries between the arts therapies merged stemmed from our history of guarding specialist boundaries. Indeed, sometimes borrowing from another modality was actually hidden, like a guilty secret. The influence of the ideas that I brought from IATE led to the team of clinicians starting to become more open about the intersection between art forms and, more importantly, to the usefulness of this for our clients.

Case vignette 1: the Crisis Café

These integrative arts approaches were also evident in our engagement in the Crisis Café, which was established in 2016 to reduce pressure in a busy A&E department. It offered an informal space for beverages and conversation with rooms off the lounge where clients could be offered brief psychological interventions, including arts therapies, to de-escalate.

We rapidly found that engaging with people in crisis necessitated a flexible approach, which used the widest possible range of tools. This meant working across arts modalities, offering whatever the situation demanded. For example, a person arrived having a panic attack and feeling suicidal and was so distraught she couldn't sit down. However, whilst they were talking, the therapist put her hand in the sandtray and started to sift the sand in rhythm with the client's speech. This had a calming effect and she sat down and joined in with the sifting. As her breathing steadied, she began to self-regulate and found an object in the tray to represent how she was now and another for how she wanted to feel. This enabled the therapist and the client to create a crisis plan.

The sifting of the sand can be seen as an invitation to engage in co-created play, similar to the kind that occurs between the infant and the caregiver. The intervention may have been effective because the client, at this point, needed to regress and be nurtured. Trevarthen (1983: 139) has described the infant–carer interaction as a "proto-conversation", a complex dance between the infant and the caregiver consisting of "synchronised (movements) . . . with gentle but rhythmic vocalisations", an important point emerging from Trevarthen's work is that infant play involves musicality, dance, and speech and is therefore multi-modal. As the example illustrates, play was often an important element in our work with clients in crisis and it is in play that the boundaries between the different arts therapies start to dissolve.

Case vignette 2: mixed modality group work

Another important development was mixed modality group work. For example, I co-facilitated a group with a dance movement psychotherapist for clients with severe depression, trauma, and medically unexplained physical symptoms.

Following the IATE approach of graded engagement (Zinker, 1978), the group started with the relatively safe ritual of clients choosing a postcard, an image, or an object to connect to the group and express how they felt. They would then do gentle body awareness work, leading to improvised movement to music, sometimes using dramatic props. Group members then transferred their movements into art making before concluding with a verbal discussion.

What was fascinating was how this mixed modality structure provided an opportunity for clients to develop and transform a motif. For example, Tina (all names have been changed to preserve anonymity), who had severe depression and medically unexplained physical pain, chose a red and black postcard image, sparking a memory of what her intestines looked like in a recent medical check. In the movement phase of the group, she felt stiff and described a sensation of having a heavy hard mass inside her. She found that she was able to jiggle this mass around slightly and this seemed to release something. Transferring this sensation into art making, she painted the hard mass as a rock and then added a red and black volcano around it. In the verbal part of the session, she identified this as her repressed anger. It is notable that the process facilitated different forms of self-expression, which did not come together in a fully articulated form until the end of a journey through different modalities.

Lacan's (1998) theoretical model involving three Registers: the Real, the Imaginary, and the Symbolic can help illuminate this journey. Notably, Lacan is not a prominent part of British arts therapy training, and I encountered his work much later in my career but found it to be helpful in understanding the value of mixed-modality practice. Lacan argued these Registers intersect each other like a type of knot known as the Borromean Knot (Figure 2.1). Each Register is also linked to a stage of infant development (Van Pelk, 2000). For the newborn infant, the world is close to the Register of the Real in that it exists as fragmented sensations and body needs, which are not yet formed into images or symbols. During the mirror phase, the child sees itself reflected in the expressions of others and forms a unified image of itself. This consolidates the child's Imaginary Register. Later, the child links images to symbols and enters into the Symbolic Register, a shared space of social meaning.

Using this theory, we can see Tina's journey of transforming a motif across art forms as a movement across three Registers. In the beginning, Tina was closest to the Register of the Real, in that she experienced fragmented, undifferentiated sensations. Through bodywork, the sensations crystalised more clearly into the image of a hard heavy mass and she began to move further into the Imaginary Register. The image was developed during the art-making phase when the rock became a volcano. Finally, reflecting on the image and discussing it with the group seemed to enable Tina to enter the Symbolic Register by seeing the volcano as a symbol of her repressed anger.

Notably, in Lacan's view, we are constantly moving between the interfaces of all three Registers (Bailly, 2009), and this suggests that therapeutic structures do not need to follow a linear sequence. Indeed, it would be more accurate to describe our mixed modality group as following a circular, rather than linear structure. In the beginning, members ritualised their entry into the group symbolically, by choosing an object or postcard to represent themselves. This proved more effective than going directly into movement work. What emerged from our circular structure was that the images and symbolic connections at the end echoed those at the beginning but were more developed. This suggested a transformation had occurred, for example, the client's image of intestines at the start of the group has the same colour scheme (red and black) as the later image of the volcano, but the image lacks the aspects (fire and rocks) that would enable her to symbolise it as anger. Our journey through the Registers is illustrated in Figure 2.1. Using different theories, one can consider this experience in different ways. Another way we could view this process is as a journey from the body to what Winnicott (1992) described as the transitional space, a space between the subject and the outside world, which is filled by the imagination. In Gestalt terms, we could view the journey as being partly about the formation of a figure by establishing a ground in body sensations (Perls, Hefferline and Goodman, 1994).

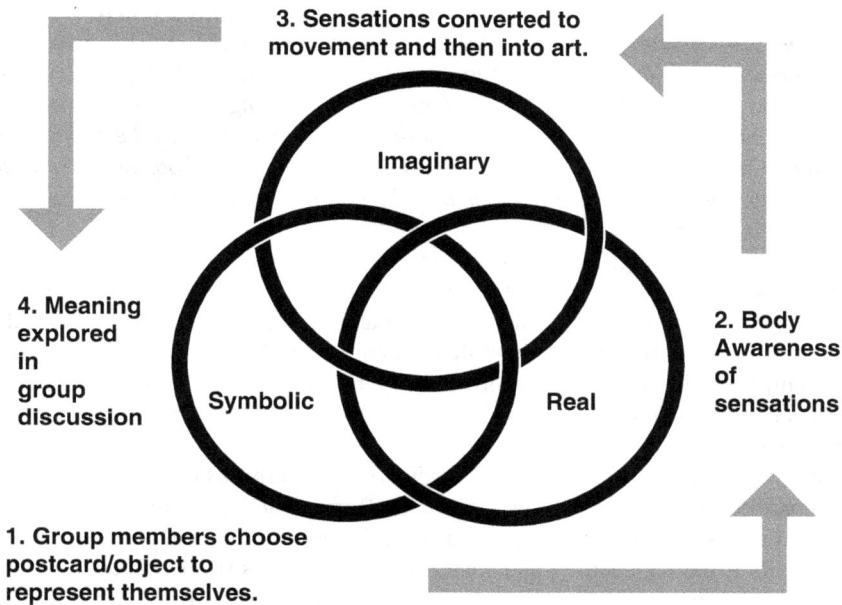

3. Sensations converted to movement and then into art.

Imaginary

4. Meaning explored in group discussion

Symbolic   Real

2. Body Awareness of sensations

1. Group members choose postcard/object to represent themselves.

Figure 2.1 A mixed modality arts psychotherapy group viewed through the lens of Lacan's Registers – a Borromean Knot (Lacan, 1998: 123–136). Image created by M. Behm

Figure 2.1 illustrates one way of sequencing a journey working across arts modalities. At times, other sequences were used, for example, in my individual work within the Department, I would sometimes start with image making and then go into a movement response to the image or the other way round, depending on how people arrived at the session and what we thought together as needed. The following case vignette illustrates this approach. As McNiff has said, "we are agents who move and change the materials and help them find a significant relationship to one another" (McNiff, 1998: 38).

Case vignette 3: individual mixed modality work

Danni had severe depression and anxiety and came over as a young adult from a war-torn country; she would often talk about her body feeling numb. She was comfortable and articulate in talking about her experiences, but her words seemed disconnected from her body. Bodywork led to the emergence of what looked like a figure-of-eight motion or movement. When I invited her to transfer this into an image, she began by making big sweeping gestures over a large piece of paper; she then made the same gesture with brushes and paint making it visible. A long stem appeared with two circles. She reflected that, by painting the figure, she had strong memories of losing a friend at 8 years of age and felt lost and abandoned with her family unable to comfort her. She began filling in the left side with staccato dots. She seemed to be struggling to find words. I asked her if there was a movement she wanted to make in response to her painting. She stroked the stem gently commenting that the dots were not dots anymore and joined them up with a paintbrush. Then she said the circles needed to be balanced, choosing to transfer the colours on one side to the other thereby creating a harmony she seemed to have been seeking.

What is interesting about this example is that Danni's figure-of-eight motif was worked with over many sessions through her stepping inside and outside her body using an approach that offered both art and movement work, woven closely together. There is something about this interweaving of art forms that led Danni to identify so closely with the motif that she became the image, stroking it as a means of self-soothing. The connecting of the dots within felt like a greater connectedness between the parts of herself.

We might see this interconnectedness in Lacanian terms as being about joining the connections between the Registers in the Borromean knot. Arguably, the subject or self is situated in the knot, and hence this weaving together of the Registers is vital to us having a strong and clear sense of ourselves (Bailly, 2009). We can see the Registers intertwining in the client's journey. For example, the figure of eight was both a physical movement and symbolic of being 8 years old and an image of a flower. Notably, at points of integration, Danni also reported a feeling of harmony and balance. Reflecting back on her work, she said later that she would not have been able to achieve this sense of balance and integration without combining art forms.

What also seems to have been particularly important in the client's journey is the connection between the body and the image that was created by the blending of artwork and movement. There is a strong parallel between this and the integration that takes place at the mirror stage of infant development, described by both Winnicott and Lacan, where the infant sees itself reflected in the gaze of others and is able to develop an image of its own body as a whole entity rather than a fragmented mass of sensations (Lacan, 2006; Winnicott, 1971; Kirshner, 2011). As the existentialist philosopher Merleau-Ponty put it:

> Visible and mobile, my body is a thing among things, it's caught in the fabric of the world, and its cohesion is that of a thing. But, because it moves it self and sees, it holds things in a circle around itself.
>
> (Edie, 1964: 163)

The arts therapies are a useful way of working with people who find it difficult to articulate their thoughts. Whilst verbal articulation is usually a vital part of arts psychotherapy work, the arts therapy process is also more than this. It allows the client, through using things like gestures, the weight of mark, a rhythm, to communicate parts of the "knot" of the self that they can't yet put into words. As the aforementioned example illustrates, the client's sense of self can be strengthened by a combination of what is articulated and what is shown. Using a variety of non-verbal modalities can enrich the communication and through this shared experience, the client's sense of self.

Mixed modalities and the therapeutic relationship

Central to any successful arts psychotherapy process is the therapeutic relationship. As discussed, in the early days of my career, I was influenced heavily by psychoanalytic object relations theory. This was the theoretical approach that underpinned my training and the links in my work between the art psychotherapists and the psychoanalytic therapies. In these early days, there was no pressure to end therapeutic treatments, which sometimes lasted several years. Furthermore, sessions would be largely unstructured with the therapist often stepping back to provide a blank screen for the client's transference and projections.

Pressures within the NHS to increase access to clients meant that the team was encouraged to deliver shorter treatments, in a wider range of settings (such as the crisis pathway). This resulted in us adopting a more integrative range of relational theoretical models to underpin and inform our practice. For example, Clarkson's five-part integrative model (2003) combines the transference relationship with other therapeutic relationships. This was later updated by Gilbert and Orlans (2011) to include the "representational relationship", which encourages active reflection on and engagement with culture and difference.

As our work in the team developed, we found that we needed to work within a shorter time frame. This meant we needed to engage clients more immediately, and as a result, the therapist became more active in inviting the client to explore different art forms as part of a co-creative relationship (Gilbert and Orlans, 2011). I think this made us more receptive and responsive to what clients needed. Initially, the co-creative space is "a working alliance" in which the therapist and the client agree to work together across different art forms. Then once they enter into the art making, co-creating becomes a more "liminal" space, in other words, an in-between space, which incorporates elements of play and where transformation can take place (Turner, 1974). Winnicott described this space as an "intermediate area of experience" (1971: 2) where play takes place and where the boundaries between me and not me become merged. In Clarkson's model, this is the "person-to-person" relationship, where "our inner and outer experience are intimately interrelated and co-existent" (Gilbert and Orlans, 2011: 69).

A strength of Clarkson's model is that it integrates a co-created approach, with a transferential approach. In our practice, making sense of transference and countertransference responses continued to be an invaluable means of understanding what clients were communicating and being able to offer a safe containing therapeutic space. Clarkson's model also fits the many-layered complexity of working across different art forms. This can be illustrated by returning to Danni's case vignette.

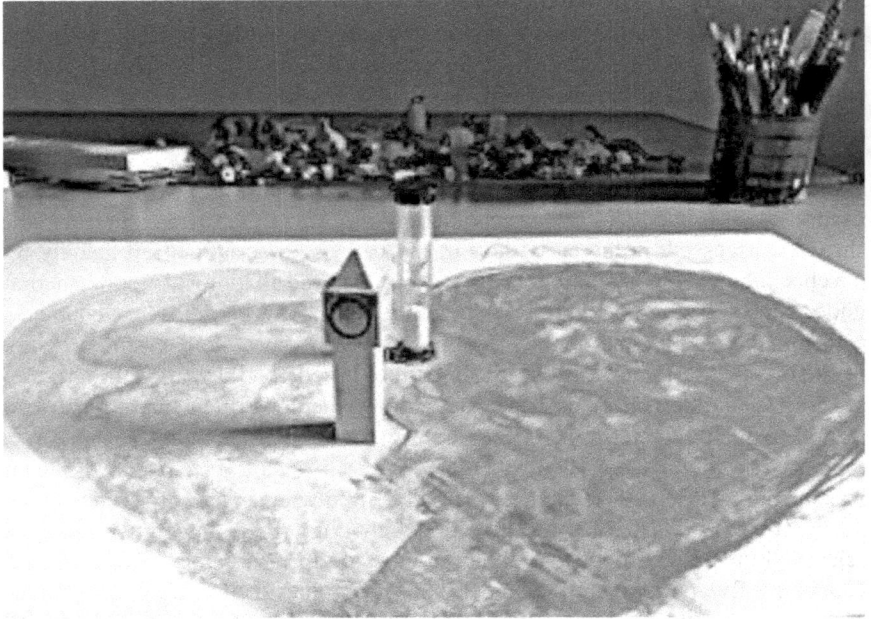

Figure 2.2 Danni's transformation of the motif

In the final months of therapy, we began our session as usual, with co-created body awareness work. Danni again returned to her figure-of-eight motif. Moving into pastels, she transformed the figure into a heart divided into a red half (labelled "anger") and a blue half (labelled "peace"), with a merged purple boundary. She then selected two objects connected to time: an hourglass and a model of Big Ben (Figure 2.2).

A heart divided into two halves is drawn on white paper using chalk pastel. One half is red with the word anger written above; the other is blue with the word peace written earlier. The colours meet in a jagged line of purple in the middle of the heart. An hourglass and a model of Big Ben have been placed alongside this line. The art materials rest on the table beyond.

In transference terms, we might associate the masculine shape of Big Ben, with her idolised but often frightening father, and the feminine shape of the transparent hourglass with her invisible mother. Looking at this together, we were able to explore how both these "time" roles were projected onto me, as the person who was responsible for bringing the therapy to an end. In addition, seeing that she had placed the objects far apart in a way that seemed to enforce the splits within her, I invited her to engage in a role play asking: "if Big Ben and the hourglass represented parts of you where would you place yourself?"

She positioned both objects close together in the liminal purple space in the centre of her image and was able to explore the objects as both "other" and part of herself. For example, she associated Big Ben with England – a country she migrated to, but with a foreign culture, which, like her father, she both idolised and found terrifying. However, in the liminal purple space, she was now also able to identify with Big Ben and her desire to achieve her own power and recognition. In Lacanian terms, the "Other" is both outside the subject, but also, as the subject seeks love from the Other, it can form part of the subject's desire (Bailly, 2009). Furthermore, whilst the Other is initially formed through the child's relationship with its primary caregiver, it is further structured by other relationships and also the surrounding culture with its networks of meaning (Bailly, 2009).

In the multi-cultural inner-city environment where I work, making sense of the client's relationship to the surrounding culture and their cultural identity is as important as working transferentially with their early childhood relationships. Furthermore, I have found that the co-created interplay between art forms enables the client and the therapist to have space to explore issues of cultural identity, through a variety of relationships. Central to this is a co-created liminal space, where the positions of me and not me can be explored and reversed.

Conclusion

I started this chapter with my memory of chasing something outside of myself – a mirage of dancing figures. These felt as if they were a part of me and connected to my moving body. This memory and my subsequent engagement with these experiences and what they might mean seemed to set in motion a dialogue, which has shaped my career and has sustained my energy for my work. IATE provided a framework, which gave me permission to pursue my interest in transforming a motif across art forms.

In clients, who have engaged in integrative arts psychotherapy, I can trace a similar pathway. They too have often taken a motif on a journey between art forms and in and out of their body. This process could link back to the formation of the subject in the mirror phase, which is experienced both as something embodied and also as an image mirrored back from outside through other people's responses to the infant (Lacan, 2006: 93). Moving between arts modalities seemed to help us to knit images and embodiment together.

Furthermore, because different arts modalities foreground the body, image, symbolisation, and role in different ways, integrative arts approaches help weave together physical sensations and symbolisation, making our motifs and our sense of self more coherent. Of course, I never reached my motif, because I was chasing a mirage, but this did not matter. It was the journey, not the arriving, that has propelled me forward to engage with the world and my imagination. In a similar way, what seems to be important, for clients I have worked with, is not fully articulating the motif or even assimilating it. Rather, it is the recognition that it is in a liminal space, both inside and just out of reach, and the sense that a striving is being set in motion, that stimulates thinking, discussion, exploration, and a re-engagement with life.

Across this chapter, I have shared a 25-year historical journey of an arts psychotherapy service. I have described how, in response to developments in practice and pressures on the NHS, we moved from operating in specialist silos to an integrative arts approach. The forces which drove us towards an integrative approach have not diminished: the pressure on crisis pathways and A&E continues, driving the need for flexible approaches, which connect mind and body; the demand for complex psychological trauma outstrips NHS therapeutic capacity, and innovations in neuroscience supporting integrative approaches, which work across mind and body, continue to develop (Porges, 2017).

Furthermore, responding to the demands of the C19 pandemic, which, at the time of writing, we are still in the middle of, requires an adaptative approach. To create social distancing, some groups now take place outside such as the Eco-Arts Psychotherapy Group. In this open space, both the therapists and the clients report that it feels natural to bring body and image together, a finding that for me resonates with my own childhood in the Australian outback.

References

Bailly, L. (2009) *Lacan.* Oneworld Publication.

Clarkson, P. (2003) *The Therapeutic Relationship.* Whurr Publishers.

Edie, J. (1964) *Maurice Merleau-Ponty: The Primacy of Perception and Other Essays on Phenomenological Psychology, the Philosophy of Art History and Politics.* Northwestern University Press.

Gilbert, M. and Orlans, V. (2011) *Integrative Therapy 100 Key Points and Techniques.* Routledge.

Kirshner, A. (2011) *Between Winnicott and Lacan, a Clinical Engagem*ent. Routledge.

Lacan, J. (1998) *The Seminar of Jacques Lacan: On Feminine Sexuality, the Limits of Love and Knowledge. Book XX Encore 1972–1973.* Trans. Bruce Fink. WWW Norton and Co.

Lacan, J. (2006) *Ecrits.* Trans. Bruce Fink. WW Norton and Co.

Lowenfeld, M. (2005) *Understanding Children's Sandplay: Lowenfeld's World Technique.* Academic Press.

McNiff, S. (1998) *Trust the Process – An Artists Guide to Letting Go.* Shambala Boulder.

Parsonage, M. and Fossey, M. (2011) *Economic Evaluation of a Liaison Psychiatry Service.* Centre for Mental Health.

Payne, H. (1992) *Dance Movement Therapy: Theory and Practice.* Routledge.

Perls, F., Hefferline, R. and Goodman, P. (1994) *Gestalt Therapy, Excitement and Growth in the Human Personality.* Blackwell.

Porges, S. (2017) *The Polyvagal Theory.* W.W. Norton and Company.

Rothchild, B. (2000) *The Body Remembers: The Psychophysiology of Trauma and Trauma Treatment.* W.W. Norton and Company.

Trevarthen, C. (1983) 'Emotions in infancy: Regulators of contracts and relationships with persons.' In K. Scherer and P. Ekman (eds) *Approaches to Emotion.* Lawrence Erlbaum Associates, Inc.

Turner, V. (1974) 'Liminal to liminoid, in play, flow and ritual: An essay in comparative symbology.' *Rice University Studies*, 60, no. 3.

Van der Kolk, B. (2014) *The Body Keeps the Score, Mind Brain and Body in the Transformation of Trauma*. Penguin.

Van Pelk, T. (2000) *The Other Side of Desire, Lacan's Theory of the Registers*. State University of New York Press.

Winnicott, D. (1971) *Playing and Reality*. Penguin.

Winnicott, D. (1992) *Through Paediatrics to Psychoanalysis, Collected Papers*. Karnac Books.

Zinker, J. (1978) *Creative Process in Gestalt Therapy*. Vintage Books.

Part II

Ideas that help us to understand the use of the arts in psychotherapy and to work integratively

Chapter 3

Integrating theory and practice

A literature review of the arts in psychotherapy

Gary Nash

Introduction

This chapter provides a review of some key theories, methods, and approaches used in the different arts therapies and places a focus on the overlaps and commonalities that can lead to an integration of the arts in psychotherapy. Although the term "integrative arts psychotherapy" is relatively new, the principles of integration have a longer history emerging from the growing field of "expressive arts therapy" which I will explore in the first section.

The second section focuses on the intersubjective relational space in which art and creativity are shaped, shared, and interacted with in therapy. The concepts of the triangular relationship and the therapeutic "third" provide a framework within which a collaborative, creative exchange can develop through the therapist's attunement and visual empathy towards the client's creative presence. The subjective experiences of both client and therapist are considered in relation to the part that the body plays in generating creative responses and is developed in the third section. This is followed by theories relating to the experience of witnessing in the arts therapies, exploring how witnessing extends the cycle of creativity, providing a meeting point in which creativity is reflected, amplified, and interpreted.

An integrative arts approach uses a range of visual, kinaesthetic, and verbal means of communication to explore, engage, and examine the art object or creative expression produced during therapy. The final section will examine how integrative arts psychotherapy utilises these different expressive modes in a graduated and experiential way that is collaborative and firmly grounded within the developing therapeutic relationship.

Integrating the arts in psychotherapy

An integrative use of the arts in psychotherapy has developed and gained prominence through the pioneering training delivered by the Institute of Arts in Therapy and Education (IATE) in London over the past 30 years. The theoretical frame, methods, and approaches used are described by integrative arts practitioners in the chapters in this book. The only previously documented account of an integrative

DOI: 10.4324/9781003155676-6

approach in Britain prior to this publication appears in the Searle and Streng edited book *When analysis meets the Arts* (2001). The chapter written by IATE trained integrative arts psychotherapist Jocelyn James describes her practice using a humanistic approach, rooted within the tradition of Jungian psychology, and reflects a particular theoretical frame used at the time. The development of a wider theoretical base along with the publication of research, theory, methods, and approaches used has occurred outside Britain at Lesley University in Massachusetts and the European Graduate School, (EGS) in Switzerland.

The grounding principles of arts integration were first formulated as the result of the creative collaboration between Shaun McNiff and Paolo Knill at Lesley in the 1970s and 80s as described by McNiff (2009), Levine and Knill (2012), and Estrella (2005). McNiff's work exploring the healing potential of using different arts media has been methodically documented. McNiff first wrote about the importance of developing an integrative perspective in *"The arts in psychotherapy"* (1981), in which he established a clear theoretical structure and approach using all of the arts in therapy. Further publications have refined the philosophical rationale and methods used; these include *"Pantheon of creative arts therapies: An integrative perspective"* (1987), *"Art as Medicine"*, (1992) and *"Art Heals"* (2004). The term "expressive arts therapy" was first introduced by McNiff (1981) as using a combination of different modes of expression: *"the expressive therapies of art, dance, drama, music and poetry have an essential unity and complement each other in practice"* (p. viii) and that by allowing a full range of creative arts expression: "we augment the clinical depth and scope of the arts" (p. viii). His work has been at the forefront of the development of Expressive Arts Therapy and is described in *"Integrating the arts in therapy: History, theory and practice"* (2009). The formulation of using an integrative approach in research was also established by McNiff with the publication of *Art based research* in 1998. The theoretical exploration of the integration of the arts in therapy is also described by Knill, Barba, and Fuchs *"Minstrels of the soul: Intermodal expressive therapy"* (1995). The transitions within and between artistic modalities are examined through Knill's 'intermodal' model and polyaesthetic theory. Prior to this publication art therapist Arthur Robbins (1994) published *A multi-modal approach to creative art therapy* in which the movement between art modalities is conceptualised using a theoretical framework which draws from object relations, ego psychology, and psychological aesthetics.

The practice of combining different arts media, methods, and research that began in the 1970s emerged as a distinct discipline in the 1990s with the establishment of the International Expressive Arts Therapy Association (IEATA) in 1994. The umbrella term "expressive arts therapy" was adopted and defined drawing on the work of McNiff (1981, 2004), Knill et al. (1995), Levine (1997), and Levine and Levine (1998). A central theme shared by the expressive and integrative arts therapies is in working with the interconnections between various art forms and media. McNiff (2004) describes how the arts can be experienced as holding an integrative potential by removing the conceptual demarcations imposed when differentiating media and form. By allowing the arts to work together art therapy can enable a "total expression", allowing the "free flow of creative energy within the process of healing" (p. 147). McNiff (1981, 2004) and Knill et al. (1995) describe the importance of the unifying experience of creativity and how the different art forms support connection to feeling, the expression of internal affects, and the creative experience that connection and expression enhances.

In the publication *Expressive arts therapy* (2005), Malchiodi describes how using more than one creative art form is based on an understanding that each art media, method, and process have unique properties that contribute to the therapeutic needs of the individual, depending on the context, the therapeutic relationship, and material being worked with. She offers a definition that highlights some of the characteristics of expressive arts therapy including: "self-expression; active participation; imagination and mind-body connections" (p. 9). The expressive arts and integrative approach value equally an attention to the sensory process of creative expression and the shared experience of the creative artwork, objects, poetic expression, sound improvisation, enactment, or visual narratives that emerge.

A theoretical understanding of the integration of the different art forms and the key concepts within art, drama, music, dance and movement, and body-oriented therapies, will equally inform the literature review in the next section. The aim is to consider the interconnected nature of the arts in psychotherapy and the overlaps between visual, performative, and dramatic arts.

Verbal, non-verbal, visual, and linguistic communication

A core element within all arts therapies training involves the study, research, and understanding of language in its various forms alongside the communicative properties of the visual and performing arts. This principle is based on increasing the practitioner's sensitivity and attunement towards the subtle ways in which people express themselves and communicate ideas, emotions, and identity through verbal and non-verbal expression. The centrality of communication, both discursive and non-discursive, literal and symbolic, has informed research and theory across all the arts modalities and provides an epistemological area of discovery that continues to inform learning and practice.

In a psychotherapy context, linguistic forms of communication may, at an intrinsic level, be framed as a narrative telling of one's "story". Every client has their own personal and unique story that describes a biographical, social, political, historical, and cultural lifeline of events, relationships, hardships, losses, and traumas. Edwards (1999) places the processes of narrative central to therapy: "Image-making, story-telling, therapy and research are each, in their own way, concerned with joining actions, intentions, emotions, perceptions and events into meaningful narratives though these narratives may take on different forms" (p. 7). When an art media or creative arts method is introduced into the psychotherapy relationship, there is an opportunity to engage with a range of non-verbal, arts-based narratives.

They may complement the verbal stories we tell, and they also have the potential to expand and deepen our personal narratives.

Verbal, visual, and performative storytelling is given texture and feeling through the interactive flow between memory and imagination. The use of mental imagery or thinking in images can come naturally to some, and the use of metaphor can be used to widen the range of images evoked. Dramatherapist Sue Jennings (1990) describes storytelling as having several elements that are considered central to dramatherapy practice: "we do not just tell the story as a verbal reportage, we dramatize it; we embody it; project it and enter into role with a number of variations in the drama" (p. 17). Jennings describes the use of dramatic enactment of the story by using projective play, role play, and the use of the body, viewing dramatherapy as an embodied action-oriented process.

Metaphoric narratives and the arts

In verbal psychotherapy, the use of metaphor is a creative cornerstone through which the client's most potent life experiences are approached indirectly. Metaphor literally means to carry over and is used to "describe one thing in terms of another so that from this comparison a 'third thing', the new idea, is born" (Siegelman, 1990, p. 4). According to Siegelman (1990), metaphor underpins creativity in language development and is also reflective of an embodied experience: "metaphor, the basic way of increasing our understanding, uses body experience as the vehicle through which it reaches out to non-body experience, just as an artist uses physical media – clay, paint, metal, stone – to evoke non-physical ideas, visions or states" (p. 24). In his book entitled *The role of metaphor in art therapy: Theory, method and experience* (2007), Moon describes how metaphor supports the exploration of difficult material within the therapeutic relationship: "Metaphoric stories are often ambiguous and indirect, holding potential for multiple interpretations. By virtue of these attributes, metaphors may help therapists develop positive therapeutic alliances by avoiding negative reactions to more overt confrontations" (2007, p. 10). In psychotherapy, metaphor provides a linguistic bridge through which we can explore and relate to internal feeling states and gain access to the rich, deeper seams of the imagination, where words and images are used to connect seemingly paradoxical experiences. Stern (1998) describes the importance of the "key therapeutic metaphor" that emerges in psychotherapy and is used to bring understanding and change in the client's life: "this experience can be called the 'narrative point of origin'" (p. 257), "Most therapists would agree that one works with whatever reconstructive metaphor offers the most force and explanatory power about the patient's life, even though one can not get at the 'original edition' of the metaphor" (p. 257).

The visual and performing arts expand the potential of the therapeutic use of metaphor by giving shape, colour, form, and movement to the client's metaphoric narrative. Each creative art form has its own distinct qualities that can resonate with and amplify the client's story: Music, sound, and rhythm can activate the mood, sensation, and memory of significant metaphoric narratives; the visual arts provide graphic forms, textures, and imagery that can tap into imaginal and abstract metaphors that are multileveled or may hold multiple representations, whilst the dramatic arts develop metaphoric storylines through using movement, props, projection, and role-play to embellish and embody the characters and drama within the narrative.

Art-based expression and symbolic speech

The principle of externalising internal experience through the arts is a therapeutic process that is described by all the creative arts therapy theories (Levens, 2001; Jones, 2007). According to Skaife (2008), art conveys something about the client's lived experience as seen through the eyes of the client and externalised through the artwork. The experience of being with the client's creative process and seeing an image made gives a time and space context. Skaife argues that art is also a performance and acts as a hinge between words and images, between the imagination and the sensory experience of art making. Jennings (1990) and Skaife (2008) use the term embodiment in this context, linking the language of the image, as well as the act of making it, to communicate something about the client's lived experience. Dance and movement therapist Penfield (2001) draws a comparison between visual arts and body movement: "In artistic expression, the material may not become verbally conscious, but it does become visible to the external world" (p. 110). In movement therapy, the same phenomenon occurs: "the emotional dynamic may become visible through movement qualities, but the experience behind the movement may not be verbally described" (p. 110). Thus, the arts hold, contain, and make visible the internal experience of the client, to be seen and witnessed through the ability of the arts to give expression to feeling using "symbolic speech", as first described by Naumburg (1966).

Music therapist Odell-Miller (2001) describes a creative and philosophical tension between the art form, the dynamic human relationship, and the translation of sound into words. The same tension has shaped the theories and practices of visual arts therapy as theorists and educators shift the focus of attention from the art-making process to the art object created, from the articulation of the experience to locating meaning within the image. The resulting theoretical dichotomy alternates between the inherent healing that takes place when we are actively creating music or art (Lee, 1992; McNiff, 1992, 2004), the importance of a verbal articulation of the process (Robbins, 1994; Maclagan, 2005; McNiff, 2004), and the verbal interpretation of the symbolic value, metaphoric language, and psychological meaning within the composition or image (Stewart, 1996; Maclagan, 2001). Music and art therapy share the same theoretical principles that seek to examine how the creative act is healing and how, as specialist practitioners, we hold, shape, and facilitate the creative expressions of those we work with.

The conceptual frame provided by theories relating to the triangular relationship and the therapeutic third will help locate the central position of creativity as it occurs within the therapeutic relationship.

Between art and relationship: intersubjectivity and the therapeutic space

The triangular relationship and the therapeutic "third"

In art therapy theory, the triangle relationship is described as containing a complex range of dynamic expressive potential that contribute to, and further the process of communication, creative engagement, and therapeutic change (Schaverien, 1990, 1992, 2000; Case, 1990, 2000; Wood, 1990). The three conceptual points of the triangular relationship are described as a) the intersubjective world of the client, b) the creative, expressive acts, art works, imagery, and objects accessed, shaped, and given form during the therapy, and c) the observing, witnessing, and interactive presence of the therapist. The artwork is often seen as the creative surface upon which the collaborative focus of both the client and the therapist come to rest, to examine, absorb, explore, and seek meaning; however, each dynamic part of the triangular relationship also influences, shapes, and affects the others in a relational cycle of creative energy. The oscillation of the creative cycle between a client and their image generates a subtle energetic ripple that is contained within the triangular relationship, and which activates a wider energetic field. Case (2000) revisited the simplicity of the triangular shape arguing for "more complex forms to match the multiple and refracted projections within the art therapy room" (Isserow, 2008, p. 35). Subsequently, the triangular relationship is constantly open to emotive, affective, and creative stimulation as each new artwork is created or as each new feeling or unspoken affect rises in the interactive space between the client and the therapist.

Working psychotherapeutically with music, imagery, and the body gives access to an internal narrating space in which imaginative associations are facilitated and imaginal processes activated. In the creative and performing arts, the media holds an expressive potential and the created object, painting, sculpture, sandtray, or piece of music presents us with a third element, a dynamic sensory form that emerges and takes shape in the context of the triangular relationship. Music and visual art therapists have identified the "third" as the relationship between the client, their therapist, and the creative form that develops in-between. McNiff (1981):

> the artwork may be a bridge between them, a third object. . . . Which gives them a middle ground through which they can be together. For one person, the intermediary might be a drawing, for another a poem or perhaps a series of movements.
>
> (p. x111)

Expressive art therapists Eberhart and Atkins (2014) describe the qualities of the third as: "The arrival of the third opens up the dualistic relationship between client and counsellor and changes it to a threesome. And this, in turn, enriches the situation, enables new ways of communication and opens up new perspectives" (2014, p. 48).

In psychotherapy, the "analytic third" is described by Ogden (1994) as a co-constructed phenomenon that exists between two people and is amplified in the psychotherapy relationship. Ogden describes the "third" as consisting of three "subjectivities" within the therapeutic relationship, these are the therapist's inter-personal and intra-personal subjective experience of the other; the client's inter-personal, internal, and intra-personal subjective experiences of self and other, and the "analytic third" which is the intersubjective relationship that both the therapist and the client experience. The definition given by Gilbert and Orlans (2011) is that the "analytic third 'belongs' to neither therapist nor client, but rather to both of them simultaneously" (p. 153). They explain that the "third" is the co-created unconscious relationship that is a "fundamental part of any relationship between two people" and it is "co-constructed by the interaction in the dyad, and in turn influences the evolving process of both people's subjective experience" (2011, p. 153). They develop this understanding across the therapeutic relational model and link it to Bruber's relational stance: "we view the co-creation of this 'therapeutic space' as the heart of an affective working alliance. This is similar to Buber's (1923/1996) concept of the 'between' – as at the heart of dialogue in gestalt therapy" (2011, p. 154). Gerson (2004) refers to the analytic third in spatial terms as a shared space in which a certain quality of dialogue occurs: "a reflective space based on mutual recognition, and which allows therapy to take place" (p. 78). The third is therefore considered to be an imaginative and sensory response to the intersubjective experience of both participants.

The principle of externalising internal subjective affect through art enables a parallel process to occur as physiological experiences, or rises of affect, in the body of the client are expressed in the artworks as well as in the non-verbal communication between the client and the therapist. This area of intersubjectivity is defined by what the client brings into the session and is equally influenced by how the therapist responds, thus resonating with each part of the triangular dynamic as an expressive act is witnessed, absorbed, and responded to within the intersubjective experiences of both the therapist and the client. A growing understanding of empathy, attunement, and the therapist's embodied experience of intersubjective phenomena has contributed to theoretical developments in this area of practice as described in the next section.

The body, creativity, and visual empathy

Within the literature on developing an integrative approach, there are several overlapping principles that emerge. The definition given by Searle and Streng (2001) attempts to find pathways between the body, the mind, feelings, and perceptions, and Gilbert and Orlans (2011) examine the importance of the inter-relation between the physiological, affective, and cognitive behavioural systems.

A resonant theme is that of the interconnectivity that we experience as embodied beings both as therapists and for those we work with. An embodied process is active within each part of the triangular relationship through the presence of the body of the client, the use of the body to create, express or enact an arts-based narrative, and the body of the therapist, which is used to receive, respond, and relate through empathy and attunement.

A physiological theory of empathy

The connection between empathy and intersubjectivity is described by Eberhart and Atkins (2014) as one's:

> capacity for empathy is closely tied to the imagination. To experience empathy we must be able to imagine and appreciate the subjective world of the other, even though it may be vastly different from our own experience of the world.
>
> (p. 64)

Empathy in relation to the art object is examined by Franklin and Politsky (1992) in their paper on interpretation in art therapy. They explore how empathy is situated between listening and interpreting and serves as a pre-condition for both. They argue that the empathy experienced between the therapist, their client, and their artwork is an intra-psychic process whereby we develop the capacity to approach what another person is experiencing yet remain separate, reflective, and understanding. Empathy in relation to the artwork is given the term "image-centred" and expands the likelihood that the therapist will objectively connect with the visual phenomenon presented: "the orientation of empathy, it seems, is a crucial component of deciphering meaning in affectively charged artworks" (p. 166).

The centrality of visual and art-based empathy is developed further by Franklin (2010) as he defines the intersubjective experience that occurs between the therapist and the client whilst witnessing the art-making process. Franklin found that the therapist's focused attention on the art making builds attunement and increases empathic resonance: "at its core, empathy is instinctually an intersubjective, imaginal practice of entering the world of another" (p. 161). He refers to neurobiological studies of the "mirror neuron system" and considers how looking, viewing, and witnessing the creative acts of others evoke or trigger "strong visceral" responses in the viewer (p. 161). In the context of Franklin's paper, he suggests that conversely "visual conditions could be designed to cultivate forms of 'as if' resonance to serve empathic communication within the therapeutic relationship" (p. 161) when, for example, the therapist responds to group affect by making an image to reflect the empathic experience within the therapy session or when working alongside, as described by Marshall-Tierney (2014) and Havsteen-Franklin and Camarena Altamirano (2015).

Somatic countertransference

Attunement and empathic resonance experienced in the body and imagination of the therapist have a combined physiological effect that has been described as "somatic countertransference" by Bernstein (1984). The term was first used by Bernstein to define counter-transferential reactions that occur as physical and sensory experiences in the body of the therapist when working with body movement. Dance and authentic movement therapist Pallaro (2007) describes how the therapist as witness: "utilizes her somatic countertransference, including any images, feelings and sensations generated in her own unconscious, as a means of trying to understand what is being communicated non-verbally" (p. 224), and that: "the source of our empathic felt knowledge is the body" (p. 181). Gilbert and Orlans (2011) also refer to the importance of the therapist's intersubjective experiences when considering sensory reactions from a counter-transference perspective: "an awareness of the therapist's own body sensation is likely to signal key counter-transferential responses to the client" (p. 182). The contribution to theory and method enables art therapists to understand and utilise their own somatic responses to the non-verbal and implicit communication that exists between therapist, client, and creative expressive acts activated within the triangular relationship.

According to Ogden (1994), Schore (2003), Robbins (1973), and Gilbert and Orlans (2011), a physiological response can be sensed through either a tightening or release within the body of the therapist as experienced through the contact boundary between therapist and client. Schore (2003) emphasises that the "clinician's receptive orientation allows for a condition of resonance . . . that is the crescendos and decrescendos of the empathic clinician's psychobiological state in resonance with similar crescendos and decrescendos of the patient's state" (2003, p. 79). An early paper by Robbins (1973) describes this embodied process as wave upon wave of feeling and affect are experienced in the body of the therapist. Robbins reflects on his experience of this intersubjective connection with the other: "One introject subsides and another looms up – over and over again as I creatively attempt to access the distance and closeness that are required in the relationship" (p. 183). Robbins shows how affects and imagery spontaneously occur in the body and imagination of the therapist as feeling, identification, and introject after introject rises through the body fusing, from time to time, to form an internal image. This reflective resonance is highlighted by art therapists and has been developed through the work of Franklin (2010) and Pallaro (2007), contributing to a physiological theory of empathy and unconscious process.

Witnessing and co-construction of meaning: how we respond to art

The creative arts therapies share several common dynamic elements as the therapist a) witnesses a period of creativity, b) supports the client to verbalise and recount the creative phase, c) facilitates a creative response in relation to the art-work, and d) co-constructs meaning through either the translation or interpretation of the artwork.

a) Witnessing and phenomenal noticing

The experience of witnessing and responding to the creativity of others is unique in the arts therapies. McNiff (2008) describes the role of witness as being: "among the most essential components of the therapeutic relationship, perhaps even more primary than that of a guide" (p. 127). Witnessing the manipulation of art materials, experimentation with musical instruments, or the gestural expression of the human body offers a sustained period of attunement towards the creative presence of the client. Focused witnessing is based on holding openness and curiosity towards whatever creative forms may emerge and bringing one's awareness to the creative and relational phenomena (Gilbert and Orlans, 2011). Eberhart and Atkins (2014) use the term "multileveled awareness" to describe the range of focused attention required: "to be fully present means to focus attention on the other person, on oneself, on the atmosphere in between, and on the ongoing process that is emerging in the moment" (p. 70). The attention of the therapist simultaneously scans the environment and notices the "ongoing, moment-to-moment process of the encounter" (p. 71). Awareness also oscillates between the creative acts and internal responses as we absorb the creative energy (Robbins, 1973; Zinker, 1978), respond imaginatively to thoughts, ideas, and free associations (Maclagan, 2001, 2005), and tune into the somatic experiences of modulating affects in the body (Pollaro, 2007; Franklin, 2010).

b) Articulating the creative phase

Art therapist Betensky (1973) developed a practice informed theory that investigated the interaction between sensation or perception, cognition, and emotion, finding that "art and words interact in art psychotherapy, art most often preceding words, together to comprise an exercise in awareness which attains full clarity in the act of verbal communication" (p. 335). This fundamental principle is described by Holmes (2001) as a sequential process: "(1) form, (2) activity, (3) reflection by the other (the mother, the audience), (4) reinternalization of the reflection" (p. 19). Robbins (1994) describes the movement from an art-making phase to a verbal phase in which the creative process is articulated:

> The therapist's non-verbal concern may be one property of the healing experience, but that there were also clearly times when the therapist must be able to use his ego to help the patient attend, investigate, contrast; in short, to help the patient objectify his perceptions and better cope with his inner worlds.
>
> (1994, p. 15)

The implication is that there are phenomenological differences between the creative expressive phase in therapy and a reflective verbalising phase that reflects a more cognitive articulation of the process.

c) Reflection, elaboration, and dialoguing with the arts

Maclagan (2001) promotes an awareness of all the senses and the use of a "figurative language" to fully engage with artworks in art therapy. He describes viewing a painting as "wandering about" in artworks and developing an "imaginative inhabitation" of the image (2001). Maclagan (2005) uses a Jungian informed approach and the process of "active imagination" which encourages the image/s to speak for themselves. He uses the term "animation" to describe bringing the image alive to talk and relate to: "Like narratives, animation keeps us within the metaphors of the image; it doesn't attempt to translate them into something else in the way that interpretation does" (2005, p. 28). This is similar to the "dialoguing" method used by McNiff (1992, 2004, 2009). McNiff (1992) illustrates how this approach is based on the principle of "talking with" rather than "talking about" an image (p. 105). Interpretation is presented as a process of creative and sensitive interaction and response to an artwork, whereby we try to get as close as possible to the expression. Imagination and play help us discover new possibilities and relationships that transcend the usual linear explanations and analytic reductions that tend to reinforce fixity. The approach described by McNiff "promotes interaction" with different elements, figures, feelings, textures, and patterns within the artwork:

> Dialoguing with images helps us get a better sense of who they are, how they were made, and how they influence our lives. By letting the image describe its emergence, we enter into the perspectives of the medium and imagination.
>
> (p. 108)

d) Translation, interpretation, and collaboration

The therapeutic intention, when informed by psychoanalytic theories, places a therapeutic value upon talking about the creative experience and thinking about what the art expression might mean for the client. A verbal account of the artwork invariably leads to an interpretation of its symbolic language, usually with an intention of increasing our understanding of what it might have to say. Psychoanalyst Siegelman (1990) in her work on meaning and metaphor describes the process of interpretation of verbal imagery as it occurs through the client's use of metaphor: "Psychotherapy, analysis – is an interpretative art – we foster in our patients an increased freedom to construct and re-construct meanings so as to arrive at a fuller, more complex and, in some sense, a more affectively true rendering of their experience" (p. 128). Similar processes of co-constructing meaning occur at multiple levels in an art and process-oriented psychotherapy.

Franklin and Politsky (1992) developed an "image centred" approach to working with clients in order to gain a greater understanding of affective artworks arguing that: "Every viewing of an artwork is an active process of making sense of – of interpreting – to find meaning within the work of art" (p. 163) and that: "Interpretation is taken as the most meaningful phase of the interaction between the viewer and the work of art" (p. 165). An image-centred approach requires an acknowledgement of bias and lack of total objectivity of the therapist/witness. They also present a "multidimensional" approach to interpretation that is informed by the complexity of culture, social construction, and intersectionality when approaching artworks. Similarly, Eberhart and Atkins (2014) refer to a movement from surface to depth:

> In responding to art, we are careful to begin on the surface of the art product with purely descriptive responses before moving more deeply into associations and meanings, carefully avoiding quick interpretations. We let the work speak to us in its own language.
>
> (p. 77)

Interpreting does not mean fixing or defining the object or act in context; it is a process of listening, questioning, and amplifying what is already present. As art therapist Rubin (1984) reflects: "Interpretations are seen as possibilities, sometimes probabilities, but rarely certainties" (p. 192). Successful interpretations are felt, they are embodied, and they connect the object of art with the subject of the client in therapy. McNiff (1981, 2004, 2015), Knill et al. (1995), and Levine and Knill (2012) show how the therapeutic value of creativity can be heightened when we stay with the non-verbal language that originates within the body and resonates through an arts enactment. They caution against following a linear sequence that leads towards a verbal articulation of meaning describing how, if we stay with an arts-based vocabulary, we stay closer to the phenomenological experience of the client's creative expression. Rather than moving too quickly towards a verbal reasoning mode of language and the interpretation of art, they encourage practitioners to inhabit or dwell within the visual and sensory processes of the creative act, and to consider how we can use art to interpret art.

Witnessing the creative presence of others is not a static state. According to Eberhart and Atkins (2014), therapeutic and creative presence: "is also an interactive encounter with whatever is present in awareness, including the self, the other and the atmosphere that is created in the in-between" (p. 75). When we use the sensory experience of witnessing along with curiosity, multi-levelled attention, and sensory attunement, we find that the creative act touches the body and mind of the therapist. The ways in which the therapist responds to the creative presence within the triangular relationship will then be shaped by various facilitation methods. I will introduce some integrative approaches in the next section.

Integrative methods and approach

Creative experimentation

The transition between linguistic/verbal and non-linguistic/visual or non-verbal/ body language is described as "language switching" by Morrell (2011). He describes how the movement from verbal narration to internal imagery and then to embodiment or image-making is framed by the therapist's facilitation approach:

> A psychoanalytic and client-centred approach tends to use a code-switching model in which the client may switch back and forth between art and speech at will. The therapist will follow the client's lead and allow them to express themselves in whatever mode they choose.
>
> (2011, p. 30)

Therapists may use other, more directive approaches, whereby they invite a language switch by asking – "do you have an image this week?" – "what would that experience look like?" or "would you be able to draw how it feels?" This describes two common approaches used to frame an arts therapy session, with the second example giving more structure to the transition from one form of communication to another.

In integrative arts psychotherapy, the structure of a session is framed as a collaborative process of exploration and experimentation using all the arts. The term "creative experiment" is used in gestalt therapy (Zinker, 1978; Frank, 2003) and in an integrative approach, providing gradual exposure to the expressive qualities of different arts media. The "creative experiment" is defined by Zinker (1978) as: "the cornerstone of experiential learning. It transforms talking into doing, stale reminiscing and theorizing into being fully here with all one's imagination, energy, and excitement" (p. 123), and "if it works well, helps the person leap forward into new expression, or at least it pushes the person into the boundaries, the edges where his growth needs to take place" (p. 125). The therapeutic relationship provides an interactive space in which stimulation, reaction, and response of both the therapist and the client can be shared and articulated. The therapist uses her empathic and imaginative responses as the basis of the introduction of an experiment. The process of experimentation is described by Frank (2003) as "there is no specific outcome of the therapy experiment, only a moment-to-moment heightening of what is real and what is true" (p. 25).

The creative arts experience is also deeply situated in the relational exchange between both participants, and all creative experiments are mutually agreed as a different art media is suggested, or a movement or position in the studio is considered. Each experiment is also graded to varying levels of depth or intensity based on the client's choice and levels of trust and comfort. For example, a mark or gesture may be extended to gain larger sweeps or strokes on the page, and the narration of a poem may offer an opportunity to alter the volume and tone of the voice, thus amplifying or dramatising the performance. Moving from dry materials to wet paint and using fingers rather than a brush are also examples of graduated experimentation with the different language forms offered by the arts.

Creative transition between art forms

The movement from one mode of communication to another is termed "intermodal transition" by Knill et al. (1995) and Levine and Knill (2012) and provides a practice-based theory that develops the therapist's skills and knowledge in transitioning between the different arts. As a pioneer of expressive arts therapy, Knill describes the movement within art media as well as the movement between different art forms in the book *Minstrels of the soul* (Knill et al., 1995). The movement within an art process is described as an "intermodal improvisation"; however, this term is distinguished from the movement between art media which is an "intermodal transfer". Knill insisted that the experience of movement between different art media is not the focus of this approach and that:

> you don't need to do an intermodal transfer unless the work calls for it or the situation makes it necessary; nevertheless, we still work intermodally even when using one artistic discipline. This is because intermodal practice looks not only at the interface of art disciplines but is also sensitive to the mode of expression or communication within the work. It is the movement that comes through in a poem and could go into the dance or not?
> (Levine and Knill, 2012, p. 20)

The intention of "intermodal transfer" according to Knill is the movement between different ways of inquiring and experiencing, and then externalising that experience through an arts media that best resonates with the feeling. It is more about the perception and imagination of the therapist than it is about a phased or staged transition from one art form to another. Knill described film media as an example of a multi-modal experience in which the visual, compositional elements work in parallel with sound, movement, drama, and the soundtrack, to describe a scene and tell a story by using all the arts and drawing on all the senses (Levine and Knill, 2012). The film media example is used to illustrate the flow of narrative and expression in the therapy experience with the therapist receiving, absorbing, and responding to the different sensory cues.

Improvisation – responding to creative presence

The movement between different arts media requires an element of spontaneity and improvisation, framed within the structure provided by the creative experiment. The use of improvisation within the therapeutic relationship is based on attunement and developing a reciprocal process of interaction. Being touched by another's creative presence underpins an authentic response as the therapist's feelings and imagination are activated during the focused witnessing of the other. An attuned prompt, or an impromptu suggestion also requires a degree of spontaneity as well as judgement and timing. Gilbert and Orlans (2011) suggest that: "they arise in a here-and-now movement of contact out of your accumulated knowledge of the other" (p. 189), and in "good improvisation there is a sense of a fit between the therapist's intervention and the client's sense of self experience" (p. 188). A combination of spontaneity and respectful attention is based on the therapist allowing thoughts and associations to rise and take form in the imagination, to listen to the sensations in the body, and to allow the sensory experience being evoked in the moment to connect with arts-based methods of expression.

The use of artistic media to respond to creative presence provides the therapist with imaginative forms of interaction and art-based engagement that enables relationship building through art. Odell-Miller (2001) describes how music therapists use a call and response approach to interact with a client's musical composition. Authentic movement therapist Payne (1993) uses observation and attunement to respond to the client's body movement using improvisation and creative, relational movement responses. In the visual arts, Marshall-Tierney (2014) and Havsteen-Franklin (2014) show how when working alongside a client, the therapist uses attuned art making based on mirroring, copying, or following the client's directions. These methods of interaction extend the term "interpretation" by reflecting or echoing the client's creative presence within complementary arts-based expressive forms.

McNiff (2004) demonstrates how the kinetic or movement basis of visual arts provides a connective and improvisational language through which the therapist can engage, respond, and interact with a client's creativity. McNiff describes how the creative act is based on movement and that by attending to the movement, we witness how the physical gestures that form the bedrock of an artwork can open a flow of energetic creative expression through the chosen medium. This art-based interaction is termed "movement interpretation" and is developed through the physiology of touch, movement, and kinesis that creative acts require in their expression. The use of movement interpretation is an attuned, body-informed response towards the client's image, and when the therapist uses movement in return, this has the effect of amplifying the creative energy that has been activated through the art-making process. The creative cycle is completed through viewing, sharing, reflecting with, and articulating the creative arts and movement process. The verbal articulation of the experience gives voice to the energy activated in the body by resonating through the voice or by amplifying with words, journaling, or written poetry, providing a completion phase for the therapy session. Using visual, kinaesthetic, and/or verbal methods of exploration, therapists seek to engage, and examine the art object or creative expression through utilising different expressive modes of communication. The use of "art to interpret art" and "imagine the expression further" as described by McNiff (1981, 1992, 2015) builds upon the Jungian tradition of active imagination.

Conclusion

The strands that connect: integrating art, mind, and body through creative arts media

The literature review shows how creative acts and enactments in therapy have a four-part process that therapists facilitate, witness, and respond to a) the sensory, physical movements, gestures, and energetic expression that mobilises creativity, b) a reflective, absorbing, viewing, and explorative phase, c) a responsive, interactive phase in which artworks are responded to via creative extension or amplification, and d) a reflective, cognitive phase in which the experience of the previous three phases is absorbed, verbalised, and articulated. This creative cycle is witnessed by the therapist, thus bringing a wider, shared, and interactive dynamic that is met by the imaginative and responsive attunement of the therapist.

The arts therapies are distinguished from other forms of verbal psychotherapy and counselling by this unique experience of witnessing the creativity of others and it is common to all the creative and performing arts. Witnessing creative acts and expressive enactments, as this chapter shows, engages the senses, the body, and imagination of the therapist, providing a distinctly variable area of explicit and implicit communication between the client and the therapist as mediated through the creativity of both. The importance of witnessing the creative act unfold in the timeframe of an art therapy session, both individual and group, stimulates an energetic response within the therapist that resonates within the triangular dynamic relationship. Whilst witnessing an artwork being created, the movement of the client's body, or a musical improvisation, the therapist absorbs the creative expression and experiences a resonance or a physical sensation moving through the body. The physical sensation may trigger an imaginative stirring leading to a playful association through words, images, or metaphors in the mind of the therapist. This is an embodied experience whereby our imaginative process engages or plays with the visual, sensory experiences we are having in relation to the creative formation taking place before us. These body/thought sensations are accessed through reverie, imaginative associations, empathy, attunement, and bodily sense of affect modulation. An integrative theory of the triangular relationship and the therapeutic "third" emphasises the potential for subjective phenomena of both the client and the therapist to converge within the creative space in-between, through whichever art media is being used. An integrative approach considers how the therapist's facilitation of creative arts expression is shaped by the imaginative and sensory experiences occurring within this intersubjective space.

Art and creativity are experienced in a shared external space where intersubjectivity is mediated through symbolic activity. This is done collaboratively, and an integrative arts approach will use other art form narratives that respond to and interact with the original work of art. The use of the creative arts gives a space, platform, or frame within which the key therapeutic metaphoric narratives can be held and responded to through the physicality offered by the art object, enactment, or recording. The visual expression of the narrative can develop on the paper where the storylines are imagined further, elaborated, and interacted with using curiosity and dialogue. The drama of the narrative may be paused, disassembled, amplified, echoed, mirrored, or reversed, and the sound improvisation can be responded to in the call-and-response play of music. The arts enable the therapist and the client to work with the memories, projections, and potency of important metaphoric narratives through the symbolic language of creativity, art, and experimentation in the "what-if" spaces provided by the arts in psychotherapy.

References

Bernstein, P.L. (1984) The somatic countertransference: The inner *pas de deux*. In Bernstein, P.L. (ed.) *Theoretical approaches in dance/movement therapy* (Vol. 2). Dubuque, IA: Kendal, Hunt.

Betensky, M. (1973) *Self-discovery through self-expression: Use of art in psychotherapy with children and adolescents*. Springfield, IL: Charles Thomas Publishers.

Buber, M. (1923/1996) *I and thou* (translated by W. Kaufman). New York: Touchstone.

Case, C. (1990) The triangular relationship (3) The image as mediator. *Inscape Winter*, pp. 20–26.

Case, C. (2000) 'Our lady of the queen': Journeys around the maternal object. In Gilroy, A. and McNeilly, G. (eds.) *The changing shape of art therapy: New developments in theory and practice* (pp. 15–54). London and Philadelphia: Jessica Kingsley Publishers.

Eberhart, H. and Atkins, S. (2014) *Presence and process in expressive arts work: At the edge of wonder*. London and Philadelphia: Jessica Kingsley Publishers.

Edwards, D. (1999) The role of the case study in art therapy research. *Inscape: The Journal of the British Association of Art Therapists*, 4(1), pp. 2–9.

Estrella, K. (2005) Expressive therapy: An integral approach. In Malchiodi, C. (ed.) *Expressive arts therapy* (pp. 183–209). New York: The Guilford Press.

Frank, R. (2003) Embodying creativity: The therapy process and its developmental foundation. *British Gestalt Journal,* 12(1), pp. 22–30.

Franklin, M. and Politsky, R. (1992) The problem of interpretation: Implications and strategies for the field of art therapy. *The Arts in Psychotherapy*, 19, pp. 163–175.

Franklin, M. (2010) Affect regulation, mirror neurons, and the third hand: Formulating mindful empathic art interventions. *Art Therapy: Journal of the American Art Therapy Association*, 27(4), pp. 160–167.

Gerson, S. (2004) The relational unconscious: A core element of intersubjectivity, thirdness, and clinical process. *Psychoanalytic Quarterly*, 73, pp. 63–97.

Gilbert, M. and Orlans, V. (2011) *Integrative therapy: 100 key points and techniques*. Hove and New York: Routledge.

Havsteen-Franklin, D. (2014). Consensus for using arts-based response in art therapy. *International Journal of Art Therapy*, 19(3), pp. 107–113.

Havsteen-Franklin, D. and Camarena Altamirano, J. (2015). Containing the uncontainable: Responsive art making in art therapy as a method to facilitate mentalisation. *International Journal of Art Therapy*, 20(2), pp. 54–65.

Holmes, J. (2001) Freud, psychoanalysis, and the arts therapies. In Searle, Y. and Streng, I. (eds.) *Where analysis meets the arts: The integration of the arts therapies with psychoanalytic theory* (pp. 13–25). London: Karnac Books Ltd.

Isserow, I. (2008) Looking together: Joint attention in art therapy. *International Journal of Art Therapy*, 13(1), pp. 34–42.

Jennings, S. (1990) *Dramatherapy with families, groups and individuals: Waiting in the wings*. London: Jessica Kingsley Publications.

Jones, P. (2007) *Drama as therapy: Theory, practice and research* (2nd ed.). London: Routledge.

Knill, P., Barba, H.N. and Fuchs, M.N. (1995) *Minstrels of the soul: Intermodal expressive therapy*. Toronto: E.G.S. Press.

Lee, C. (1992) Stretto – the relationship between music therapy and psychotherapy: The need for professional questioning. *Journal of British Music Therapy*, 6(1), p. 23.

Levens, M. (2001) Analytically informed art therapy. In Searle, Y. and Streng, I. (eds.) *Where analysis meets the arts: The integration of the arts therapies with psychoanalytic theory* (pp. 41–59). London: Karnac Books Ltd.

Levine, S.K. (1997) *Poiesis: The language of psychology and the speech of the soul*. London: Jessica Kingsley.

Levine, S.K. and Levine, E.G. (1998) *Foundations of expressive arts therapy: Theoretical and clinical perspectives*. London: Jessica Kingsley.

Levine, S.K. and Knill, P. (2012) Longing for beauty and the work: An interview with Paolo Knill by Steven Levine. *Poiesis: A Journal of the Arts and Communication*, 14, pp. 10–25.

Maclagan, D. (2001) *Psychological aesthetics: Painting, feeling and making sense*. London and Philadelphia: Jessica Kingsley Publications.

Maclagan, D. (2005) Re-imagining art therapy. *Inscape,* 10(1), pp. 23–30.

Malchiodi, C. (2005) *Expressive arts therapy*. New York: The Guilford Press.

Marshall-Tierney, A. (2014). Making art with and without patients in acute settings. *International Journal of Art Therapy*, 19(3), pp. 96–106.

McNiff, S. (1981) *The arts in psychotherapy*. Springfield, IL: Charles C. Thomas Publisher.

McNiff, S. (1987) Pantheon of creative arts therapies: An integrative perspective. *Journal of Eclectic Psychotherapy*, 6(3), pp. 259–285.

McNiff, S. (1992) *Art as medicine: Creating a therapy of the imagination*. Boston and London: Shambhala Publications.

McNiff, S. (2004) *Art heals: How creativity cures the soul*. Boston: Shambhala Publications.

McNiff, S. (2008) Witnessing and responding to art with art. *Poiesis: A Journal of the Arts and Communication*, 10, pp. 126–134.

McNiff, S. (2009) *Integrating the arts in therapy: History, theory and practice*. Springfield, IL: Charles Thomas Publisher, Limited.

McNiff, S. (2015) *Imagination in action: Secrets for unleashing creative expression*. Boston: Shambhala Publications.

Moon, B. (2007) *The role of metaphor in art therapy: Theory, method and experience*. Springfield, IL: Charles C. Thomas Publisher, Limited.

Morrell, M. (2011) Signs and symbols: Art & language in art therapy. *Journal of Clinical Art Therapy*, 1(1), pp. 25–32.

Naumburg, M. (1966) *Dynamically oriented art therapy: Its principles and practices*. New York: Grune and Stratton.

Odell-Miller, H. (2001) Music therapy and its relationship to psychoanalysis. In Searle, Y. and Streng, I. (eds.) *Where analysis meets the arts: The integration of the arts therapies with psychoanalytic theory* (pp. 127–152). London: Karnac Books Ltd.

Ogden, T. (1994) The analytic third: Working with intersubjective clinical facts. *International Journal of Psycho-Analysis*, 75, pp. 3–20.

Pallaro, P. (ed.) (2007) *Authentic movement: Moving the body, moving the self, being moved.* London: Jessica Kingsley Publishers.

Payne, H. (ed.) (1993) *Handbook of inquiry in the arts therapies: One river, many currents.* London and Philadelphia: Jessica Kingsley Publishers.

Penfield, K. (2001) Movement as a way to the unconscious. In Searle, Y. and Streng, I. (eds.) *Where analysis meets the arts: The integration of the arts therapies with psychoanalytic theory* (pp. 107–126). London: Karnac Books.

Robbins, A. (1973). The art therapist's imagery as a response to a therapeutic dialogue. *Art Psychotherapy*, 1(3–4), pp. 181–184.

Robbins, A. (1994) *A multi-modal approach to creative art therapy.* London: Jessica Kingsley Publishers.

Rubin, J. (1984) *The art of art therapy.* New York: Brunner, Mazel.

Schaverien, J. (1990) The triangular relationship (2) Desire and alchemy and the picture. *Inscape Winter*, pp. 14–19.

Schaverien, J. (1992) *The revealing image: Analytical art psychotherapy in theory and practice.* London and Philadelphia: Jessica Kingsley Publishers.

Schaverien, J. (2000) The triangular relationship and the aesthetic countertransference in analytical art psychotherapy. In Gilroy, A. and McNeilly, G. (eds.) *The changing shape of art therapy: New developments in theory and practice* (pp. 55–83). London and Philadelphia: Jessica Kingsley Publishers.

Schore, A. (2003) *Affect regulation and the repair of the self.* New York: Norton.

Searle, Y. and Streng, I. (eds.) (2001) *Where analysis meets the arts: The integration of the arts therapies with psychoanalytic theory.* London: Karnac Books.

Siegelman, E.Y. (1990) *Metaphor and meaning in psychotherapy.* New York and London: The Guilford Press.

Skaife, S. (2008) Off-shore: A deconstruction of Maclagan and Mann's Inscape papers. *International Journal of Art Therapy*, 13(2), pp. 44–52.

Stern, D. (1998) *The interpersonal world of the infant: A view from psychoanalysis and developmental psychology.* London: Karnac Books.

Stewart, D. (1996) Chaos, noise and a wall of silence: Psychodynamic music therapy. *British Journal of Music Therapy*, 10(2), pp. 21–34.

Wood, C. (1990) The triangular relationship (1) The beginnings and endings of therapy relationships. *Inscape Winter*, pp. 7–13.

Zinker, J. (1978) *Creative process in Gestalt therapy.* New York and Toronto: Vintage Books.

Chapter 4

The six therapeutic relationships and the arts

An integrative approach to using theory, research, and the creative arts in practice

Claire Louise Vaculik and Vanja Orlans

Introduction

This chapter provides an overview of a structural framework that can be used to develop an integrative approach to art psychotherapy practice, demonstrating too some of the ways that the seven art forms (art, sculpture/clay, bodywork/movement, sand play, drama/puppetry, poetry, and music) might emerge, be understood, or used in an integrated and holistic way within this approach.

At IATE, we offer this framework to help our students to consider their client/s and prepare for the proposed shared therapeutic journey in its fullness, as it facilitates the bringing together of a relevant and wide-ranging amount of literature focusing on theory, research, and practice. The idea of using the relationship as a vehicle for an integrative framework for practice was originally proposed by Petruska Clarkson at Metanoia Institute, who wrote about a five relationship framework (Clarkson, 1990, 1995). She introduced this to students at IATE when she taught integration here in the 1990s. Over time, this was expanded and updated with a wider six relationship frame, as proposed by Gilbert and Orlans (2011).

The six-relationship framework provides a solid foundation for all of our teaching at IATE and feedback from students consistently affirms its usefulness for practice. It enables an art therapist to start to consider clients from each of the perspectives that can be present in a full and dynamic therapeutic relationship and then to use theory and research from different modalities to develop a holistic, coherent, and consistent approach to working with them, whilst using the arts and creativity in sessions. In addition, the framework supports the assessment of risk and a capacity to grade and pace the development of clinical work. The approach can also be reviewed or developed collaboratively over time, so that the work is relational, sensitive, and most useful for the client or group. An ongoing process of structured reflection using the framework can support the therapist and the client to hold in mind the fullness of the therapeutic relationship, enabling them to be present and to focus on how the arts and imagination bring this experience to life in sessions.

DOI: 10.4324/9781003155676-7

The case for an integrative stance on psychotherapy

Historically, we can discern an interest in integration that dates back to Freud and his contemporaries. For example, Ferenczi, in a review of approaches in psychoanalysis to early relational trauma, pointed to the limitations of schoolism, emphasising the need for psychoanalysts to revise technique and to take the lead from the patient (1994); Ferenczi also highlighted important learning from his patients in this regard. Key figures in the history of psychotherapy demonstrate the bringing together of different types of training and thinking. For example, Albert Ellis and Aaron Beck, the original founders of Cognitive Behaviour Therapy, had a background in psychoanalysis, as did Fritz Perls who developed Gestalt Psychotherapy within the humanistic tradition (Orlans and Van Scoyoc, 2009).

Current key figures in the field of psychotherapy integration are John Norcross and Marvin Goldfried, both of whom have made considerable contributions to research and conceptual clinical frameworks over many years. Their position is that there is much to be learned from different modalities that can improve the efficacy, efficiency, and applicability of psychotherapy (Norcross and Goldfried, 2019). They make reference to the historical ideological Cold War that they viewed as "a possible necessary developmental stage towards sophisticated attempts at rapprochement" (p. 3). However, as they point out, research results over the years demonstrate few significant differences between different therapeutic approaches. At the same time, they highlight the importance of matching a therapeutic response to the presenting difficulties and person of the particular client, highlighting responsiveness as a key issue in our work. Our position is that an integrative framework that allows for a consideration of a range of important therapeutic factors and possible responses to a client serves to broaden the practitioner's competencies in the clinical setting, enabling them to be creative, adaptable, and to offer the best service possible to the client. It reflects a holistic view of the person, who can be seen from a number of perspectives such as affectively, cognitively, behaviourally, physically, and spiritually (Lapworth and Sills, 2010).

It could be useful at this stage to draw attention to some criticisms that have been levelled at the adoption of an integrative approach. It has been suggested, for example, that a focus on integration is too wide ranging and runs the risk of missing an in-depth conceptualisation or depth of treatment. As a result, integrative psychotherapists would lack the in-depth knowledge of the psychotherapy process that comes from immersion in a "pure-form" approach. They could risk getting lost in too many options and lack the clarity that comes from one focus. A similar criticism is sometimes made of using a multi-arts approach in therapy. We believe that there is some validity to this criticism in trainings where there may be insufficient grounding in basic or over-arching psychotherapeutic principles and that this criticism can also apply in certain cases with certain clinicians. It is important that a training is rigorous and covers concepts and each of the seven art forms in depth, as well as providing a firm grounding in the application of technique, and space to consider tensions and conflicts between different approaches and art forms. However, the fact that there are many overlaps between psychotherapeutic theories and approaches and that the confusion of "jargons" that may, or may not be, referring to similar processes remains a missing focus in single modality approaches where certain concepts can be treated as fact and not even be considered to be schoolism-related jargon.

We know that in a training where integration is taught from the start, students are challenged to take up the position of there being no one truth, reflecting the tenets of post-modernism. At the same time, there is a need to understand the tensions of holding different perspectives. Students need to conceptualise at a meta-level from the beginning and evaluate differential intervention options. This is a challenging process and requires the development of sophisticated reflexive functioning, something that requires clear recognition and support from tutors and clinical supervisors. However, we also know that tutors will be imparting an important philosophical position together with a number of key ideas and principles, drawn from a wider number of sources, and that will be likely to enhance the capabilities of students as therapists. Our experience is that students tend to find the challenges more acute at the start of their training when they gaze across the wide landscape that lies ahead and take in the wide range of literature and research that will be covered in learning settings. However, our experience is that there is also excitement about covering leading-edge ideas and the creative possibilities that each of the art forms offers, together with a gradual appreciation of the focus on integration towards the end of the training, especially in the context of dissertation and viva preparation.

There has also been a suggestion that a focus on integration could be seen as grandiose with an implicit claim that this approach can help anyone with any problem. In response to this criticism, we would underline the position that, above all, it is vital that all therapists, integrative psychotherapists equally, know the limits of their competence at each developmental stage and do not make claims that are unrealistic and grandiose.

A relationship focus as a key organising principle

The choice of a focus on relationship was originally highlighted by Clarkson (1995) as reflecting the metanarrative that runs through the work of any psychotherapeutic approach. She makes the point early on in that book that "the work lies in the creative space between, in the relationship" (p. viii). Since its publication, we have seen a significant expansion of research and conceptualisations that further support this focus and enable such a perspective to include key research studies so relevant to our work as psychotherapists. However, we would like to underline that by focusing on the issue of relationship, we are not seeking to take up a binary position whereby the relationship is contrasted to the treatment method, a position that has been evident in the developing research literature over recent years. Along with such writers as Norcross and Lambert (2011), we would view the value of a treatment approach as inextricably bound to a particular relational context.

The benefit of focusing on relationship enables us to highlight the importance of process in a setting that includes the persons of therapist, client, and the artwork, the interactions between these, and the treatment formulations that might be likely to be most useful and effective for that particular frame. In our consideration of a number of relationship dimensions that operate within the psychotherapeutic setting, we would also like to make the point that these relationships are socially constructed and moving scenarios that unfold in different and complex ways over time. They include conscious, explicit, and verbal dimensions as well as non-conscious, implicit, non-verbal, and body-based levels of exchange. This presents the practitioner with fascinating and complex challenges of understanding, observing, and tracking as we negotiate different types of relating.

The six-relationships framework and the arts

The use of the arts in psychotherapy provides a rich resource for a therapist engaged with the task of explaining what therapy is at the start of the work as well as in subsequent exchanges as the relationship unfolds. Also, the use of art forms draws directly on right hemisphere functioning and allows insight and understanding into as yet conceptually unformed thoughts. An image or an apt metaphor can capture and contain the potentially inevitable ups and down of a therapeutic journey, conveying at an embodied level the complexity of these sorts of journeys of self-discovery in a manner that enables a client to grasp what the work may feel like. It can support the client to feel empowered, enabling them to take up a role as a collaborator in this unfolding process. Exploring the image or metaphor may also enable a more grounded and realistic appraisal to be carried out, collaboratively with the client, to ascertain what might be needed to ground and stabilise the client sufficiently to engage with the identified goals of therapy (Bordin, 1994). As therapy unfolds, this image or metaphor can be returned to and drawn upon, again and again, helping to contain some of the inevitable experiences of rupture, repair, and review so that they can be explored together.

In the following sections, we set out the specifics of our integrative framework with an overview of each relational position and some of the key issues reflected in each standpoint and suggest some of the many possible ways that different art forms might emerge or be used in an integrated and holistic way within this. It should be remembered that, while we offer these ideas from a differentiated position, we recognise that these relationship modalities constantly interweave with each other in the clinical setting, challenging both the therapist and the client to tease out what is happening and to work together creatively as the clinical process unfolds. Our focus is on a conceptual and practice-based overview of each relational frame, providing examples of the ways that each of these conceptualisations can be grounded in the use of art forms to enable arrival at a deepening understanding of the therapeutic process and the possibilities for achieving a successful therapeutic outcome. One final point relates to the order in which we are presenting these different relationships. We do not regard this as a fixed structure and invite the reader to move between the descriptions in any order that might feel right. Our own position was to start with issues that feature at the beginning of the therapeutic contract and end with the "person-to-person" relationship focus as this tends to represent a strong position at the end of therapy. However, as outlined earlier, there is considerable weaving in and out of different types of relationships throughout the process of psychotherapy.

The working alliance

Getting started with a psychotherapy contract is an interesting and widely researched area. Freud himself drew attention to the "pact" between the analyst and the patient who "band together" with a common goal (Freud, 1913, 1940); for Freud, the alliance was closely linked to a positive or idealised transference. Since that time, various writers have considered these issues. A widely known formulation of the working alliance was proposed by Bordin (1994) who emphasised three key components that included a respectful and friendly bond, an agreement on therapeutic goals, and an agreement on therapeutic tasks. The importance of establishing a working alliance is highlighted in different ways within different therapeutic modalities. Within the humanistic tradition, Carl Rogers (1959) highlighted six key conditions that needed to be present for therapy to be successful, which included a focus on the contact between therapist and client. From a cognitive behavioural standpoint, there is an emphasis on the importance of expertness and the trustworthiness of the therapist. Norcross (2010) describes the alliance as referring to "the quality and strength of the collaborative relationship". Horvath et al. (2011) refer to the alliance as a pantheoretical concept that emphasises the importance of *active* collaboration and consensus between the therapist and the client.

There has been a significant amount of research conducted on the working alliance that has included the development of measures that can be used to assess the strength of the alliance and the effects of a sound alliance on the outcome of the therapy (Horvath et al., 2011). Recent research has uncovered a number of complexities about the point at which the best predictor of outcome occurs. While there is an ongoing debate about this, current studies suggest that the establishment of a sound alliance between sessions 3 and 5 is an especially good predictor of a successful outcome. A number of interesting studies have also focused on the characteristics of both clients and therapists in promoting the quality of the alliance that develops in the dyad. On the client side, the focus has been on a capacity to maintain a relationship, the presence of broadly positive expectations, a capacity to engage in the therapeutic process, and the existence of psychological mindedness. On the therapist side, the emphasis is on a friendly and empathic attitude, a willingness to listen and to be interested in the development of collaboration, skill and willingness to deal with a client's negative or ambivalent feelings, and to be able to pay direct attention to the relationship as it develops. Safran and Muran (2006) draw attention to the complexities of these early negotiations since they will be both conscious and unconscious. Their focus is thus on the delicacy of these early exchanges, on the importance of an intersubjective stance, and the fact that these negotiations are likely to be revisited from time to time as the therapeutic journey unfolds, and where ruptures are more than likely to occur. Nonetheless, there does seem to be agreement that the way in which a therapeutic relationship begins is a very important consideration, an idea that generates much energetic debate among students in the training setting.

The use of art forms in the development or exploration of the working alliance might include variations of some of the following: shared mark-making to explore the embodied experience of being together. Use of the sandtray and miniatures to explore experience in the moment and insights this may hold for therapy. Inviting the client to draw a place where they feel safe – this might help both the client and the therapist to explore the issue of trust; understand more directly the client's phenomenology of "safety" in the context of their history, and agree on the boundaries of this collaborative endeavour; or highlight issues of what could be "unsafe", a useful guide for both the therapist and the client. Writing a poem or a story in a journal about venturing into the unknown; this could draw together the client's insights about how they tend to experience venturing into the unknown, identifying the resources they bring with them, where they might struggle, and ways in which both parties might offer support at certain important times.

The transference/countertransference relationship

The concepts of transference and countertransference are located in the psychoanalytic tradition and enable us to explore a number of complex implicit or unconscious processes in which all human beings engage and which appear in the clinical situation between the therapist, client, and artwork. Historically, these concepts were described in a more structural way and written about separately in the psychanalytic literature. The concept of transference refers to our capacity to bring the past into the present by displacing onto the therapist's feelings and ideas that derive from previous key figures and related interpersonal experiences in the client's life (Rycroft, 1979). It can also take the form of a client seeking identification in the present about an issue that occurred in the past – a form of projective identification. An example would be where the client splits off early grief based on the experience of abandonment and imagines that the therapist is sad (Racker, 1968; Clarkson, 1995). While Freud originally considered the issue of transference as a regrettable phenomenon that interfered with the recovery of repressed memories, he later came to view the analysis of transference as key to the therapeutic endeavour (Sandler et al., 1992).

The concept of countertransference refers to the emotional reaction of the therapist to the transference of the client. This reaction could either be experienced as a correspondence to the transference material of the client, i.e., in terms of our aforementioned example where the therapist feels the sadness of abandonment as a projected emotion, or it could also be that the therapist has had a similar back story and feels her own sadness as a result of this. It is often in the supervision setting that the complexities of a "reactive" or "proactive" response can be analysed and understood. The concept of countertransference has also had an interesting and evolving history within the literature on psychoanalysis. Many writers conveyed a strong emphasis on the issue as a danger to clinical work, whereas Paula Heimann, in her classic paper, described the countertransferential experience as a key unconscious communication that enabled the therapist to understand the deep implicit experience of the client (Heimann, 1950).

More recent perspectives on the concepts of transference and countertransference take the view that separating these issues does not make much theoretical or clinical sense and is also not supported by more recent research in the fields of affective neuroscience and interpersonal neurobiology (Schore, 2019; Cozolino, 2017). From this perspective, we prefer to take an intersubjective stance on these processes, drawing on a more relational perspective that focuses on paying sensitive attention to the interplay of both the client's and the therapist's ways of constructing meanings about the world as a co-constructed dance within a dynamic and ongoing process (Orange et al., 1997; DeYoung, 2015). This position is reflected in the literature on self-psychology, object relations, and intersubjectivity. A key clinical issue that arises from a consideration of this transferential/ countertransferential dance between the therapist and the client is the challenge of how to deal with self-disclosure of countertransferential material, an issue that requires some careful thought and considerable sensitivity to the existence of different self/age states in the client. Given the unconscious nature of these two-way communications, it is crucial that therapists develop the ability to view what is happening at many different levels of exchange. This is an issue that we pay close attention to in the training setting where the importance of personal therapy and good use of supervision is constantly highlighted.

Introducing art forms in the context of the transference or countertransference relationship expands this dynamic further, and it becomes a three-way communication. The use of the arts might include the following: working with art materials, movement, or music in a non-directive manner and attending to the way the client engages with this and the process of expressing themselves; the embodied experience of using the art materials can elicit unspoken projective material, from both the therapist and the client; and also, familiar expectations or assumptions may emerge or be expressed in the art as past experiences are used to make sense of, or navigate, the limitless possibilities offered by the creative process. These experiences may remain implicit or unspoken initially and can be contained and worked with in therapy, grading to manage risk as trust is developed. Inviting the client to think back to when they were a child and focusing perhaps on a favourite fairy tale or story. With the use of art materials, it would be possible to capture the essence of this story and the ways that this might appear in the present. The client might wish to expand on the meaning of these ideas in their journal.

In addition, a more immediate approach could be the creation of a family sculpture either through the use of natural found objects or through making a clay sculpture of each family member or influential people in their life. This could enable the exploration of the emotional dynamics and roles within their family that call out for attention. There could, for example, be an emphasis on a "theme tune" for each of them, or for the family dynamics as a whole, or on what each has taught them and the implications for their life at the present time. These issues could also be explored using the sandtray.

The developmentally needed relationship

In psychotherapy, clients have the opportunity to experience many positive dimensions of relating that may not have been available to them in childhood. There are a number of key experiences that enable a child to grow into a healthy adult. These have to do with the availability of an interpersonal context that promotes secure attachment (Beebe and Lachmann, 2014), supports the development of trust that things will work out OK, and engenders a sense of hope (Sroufe et al., 2005). Clients who come to us for psychotherapy have very often not had such positive experiences, leading them into difficulties at later points in their lives, whether in the forging of satisfying relationships with partners, parents, or children, or confidently being able to express themselves in the world. Previous conceptualisations of the developmentally needed relationship have sometimes referred to the "reparative" dimension as adding in a healing dimension to historical experiences. We are somewhat wary of the word "reparative" as we do not consider that previous experiences can in themselves be "repaired". Instead, what can happen is that the client is able to gain a new perspective on those experiences, working towards a situation where difficult early experiences do not intrude into, or define, current life situations, and where experiences from the therapy itself have created new and positive internal changes in the person of the client.

The focus on the developmentally needed relationship raises a number of interesting issues that have been highlighted both in clinical conceptualisations and in research. To begin with, there is the issue of a non-linear perspective on time. While this is not a new conceptualisation since it lies at the heart of transferential phenomena, it has taken on a more nuanced and varied form in more recent clinical writings. Within both psychoanalytic and trauma-focused literature, there has been an emphasis on the availability or emergence of different age-related self-states or parts of the client (see, for example, Bromberg, 2011; Fisher, 2017). Daniel Stern also pointed to this idea in his model of early development stages where he suggested that each stage continues alongside earlier developmental achievements (Stern, 1985). Irving Polster, writing within the Gestalt tradition, referred to the individual as "a population of selves" and highlighted the implications for the practice of psychotherapy (Polster, 1995). With these ideas in mind, the complexity of the psychotherapeutic process allows us the possibility of meeting "there and then" needs in the "here and now". The contributions of intersubjectivity theory and self-psychology also offer a number of useful conceptualisations as well as the implications of these for practice. Kohut's emphasis on the self-object needs of idealising, mirroring, and twinship are important here (Kohut, 1984), as is the notion of transferential layers where "there and then" issues operate alongside the newer self-object experiences in the therapeutic setting (Hagman et al., 2019). Empathy, verbal and non-verbal attunement, and key moments of deeper meeting between the therapist and different self-states of the client are key to the unfolding of this process in a positive way.

A focus on developmentally needed issues as outlined earlier inevitably requires an understanding of early traumatic experiences and the ways in which as human beings we defend ourselves in the face of these through the use of a range of primitive protective processes. In recent years, there have been significant developments in a research-based understanding of complex developmental trauma and ways of responding to this in the clinical setting. Writers such as van der Kolk (2014), Steele et al. (2017), and Fisher (2017) highlight the importance of understanding the different self-states of the client, including those that might pre-date language or that might be out of awareness. The therapist therefore needs to have a good understanding of brain and body processes (see, for example, Cozolino, 2017), how we deal with early challenging and potentially life-threatening circumstances, and the primitive ways in which, along with mammals, we protect ourselves from certain memories and related feeling states (Porges and Dana, 2018). One final important point is that to work with these early and complex processes, it is essential that the therapist has done enough significant personal therapeutic work that has led to a good understanding of their own young selves in ways that allows them to explore such issues with the client.

The use of art forms in the context of the developmentally needed relationship can be extremely helpful in finding a way into deeper right hemisphere-based issues, particularly when drawn on in a sensitive way that does not too quickly open trauma-related issues. In using visual art materials, the therapist might choose to sit alongside the client in order to moderate the contact and to enable the client slowly to build trust as they experience being in a relationship that is supportive and that also facilitates their own increasingly playful process of discovery. From this standpoint, there could be an opportunity to develop a body scan drawing helping the client to identify visually the different challenges they experience at an embodied level in making contact and being in relationship. This approach can also highlight possible developmentally needed experiences that might be offered within the therapeutic relationship. The use of puppets as a way to act out scenes also offers a creative approach for the client to arrive at a deeper meaningful understanding of experiences and relational issues relevant to different self-states. The sandtray and the use of miniatures can also enable both the therapist and the client to explore different self-states and related dynamics and to enable the client to begin to build a more integrated sense of self. In terms of the Polyvagal Theory and the very ancient ways that we have protected ourselves from the experience of threat, Deb Dana offers some helpful drawing exercises that can support and facilitate the movement from a dissociative state to the experience of safety (Dana, 2020).

The transpersonal relationship

The existence of issues and experiences in the life of a human being that cannot be fully understood, seen, or counted is an important consideration in psychotherapy and also represents an interesting critical position on an overly positivistic approach that is conveyed in a number of areas of psychotherapy research and reflected in the rise of experimental psychology in the latter half of the 19th century (Orlans and Van Scoyoc, 2009). We think that it is reasonable to describe the psychotherapeutic encounter as greater than the sum of its parts. Both issues of the existential encounter and "connection" feature as very prevalent in the consulting room, a reflection perhaps of both the therapist and the client searching for meaning in their lives. While the presenting challenges of the client can be conceptualised in terms of psychological difficulties, our experience is that clients tend to present with forms of "disconnection" and are deeply interested in locating themselves in something wider and more meaningful that is beyond the level of the individual person. To this extent, we can think of the psychotherapeutic journey as a collaborative spiritual undertaking.

It is interesting to track the introduction of the transpersonal into our current psychotherapeutic thinking. The idea of the "transpersonal" in psychological therapy has originally been attributed to the American psychologist and philosopher William James. However, the introduction of the transpersonal into psychology is generally associated with Abraham Maslow and his colleagues who founded the *Journal of Transpersonal Psychology* in 1969. Maslow was the founder of the humanistic psychology movement which he defined as the "third force" after behaviourism and psychoanalysis; transpersonal psychology was thus heralded as the "fourth force". At the same time, the writings of Carl Jung had brought issues of spirituality into psychoanalysis, emphasising a connectedness that he proposed pervaded humanity and that went beyond individual agency. Among his many interesting ideas, Jung highlighted, for example, the concepts of the archetypes and the collective unconscious (Jung, 1959; Knox, 2003; Papadopoulos, 2006).

Other writers have focused on bringing much older traditions into the psychotherapeutic frame that have resulted in new conceptual, clinical, and research interests. These have included Paul Gilbert's extensive publications and research on the importance of compassion and community (e.g., Gilbert and Choden, 2013; Gilbert, 2018), explorations of the interface between psychotherapy and religion (e.g., West, 2000), and the bringing together of Buddhism and psychotherapy (e.g., Epstein, 1995). John Rowan's writings also provide us with a useful overview of the different perspectives on a transpersonal approach to psychotherapy (Rowan, 2005). Carl Rogers, within the person-centred tradition, reminds us of the importance of "presence" as itself a transforming and therapeutic position, both for the therapist and for the client (Rogers, 1980). Again, we find that there is a very wide range of literature to be explored, often a daunting prospect for both trainees and experienced practitioners. We need to remember, however, that the purpose here is to meet ourselves and others fully in a form that transcends any kind of reductionism, that takes account of "the other" in a potentially non-objectified way, and that opens the way to a meeting that cannot be planned for but that can happen as a matter of "grace" (Buber, 1958). From such a perspective human life is met with, as transcending individual needs and plans, and this positions us as psychotherapists as willing to enter into the realm of the unknown and the yet to be found.

In terms of the use of the arts to explore these ideas, we recommend an open and free position with the idea of seeing what "emerges" into the therapy room. This might involve metaphors and images that are evoked for the client, that signify the whole being greater than the sum of the parts, and that highlight key issues of "connection". All of these issues can be illuminated in painting, the use of the voice or musical instruments, drawing, poetry, and the creative construction of stanzas that bring the individual into contact with a wider sense of being.

The representational relationship

In focusing on the representational relationship, we wish to highlight the significant importance of context in the field of psychotherapy and the ways in which we might become more sensitised and aware of a range of relevant social factors in our work. There is significant critical literature on the nature of psychotherapy that seeks to locate this activity itself within a socially constructed frame of reference (e.g., McNamee and Gergen, 1992; Gergen, 2009), pointing out how much of the thinking in this profession has been based on a medical and over scientised frame of reference that could potentially be harmful to a client. From this perspective, it can be argued that the process of individual and psychological reductionism leads to the locating of "problems" within the person expressed potentially as "symptoms", thus lending themselves to "the solution" of a psychotherapeutic response. We thus risk working within a language of deficiency and objectification. This has been a major criticism of a structural approach to mental health challenges, as described, for example, in the Diagnostic and Statistical Manual for Mental Disorders (2013), now in its fifth edition (DSM-5), or in the International Classification of Diseases (2021), now on its 11th revision (ICD11). There can be a tendency to see view certain descriptions as "facts" rather than as reflections of particular professional perspectives based on a range of social factors. For example, in earlier versions of the DSM, homosexuality had been described as a "disorder" and it was not until the publication of DSM-III-R in 1987 that this was dropped. Understanding this history is important, both for trainees and for qualified psychotherapeutic practitioners, while being knowledgeable about current constructions in terms of potential conversations, for example, with psychiatric colleagues. A psychotherapist might also be called upon to hold considerable tension between different perspectives in the interest of offering the best possible help to their client.

The practice of psychotherapy and the concepts and theories that inform this activity have also been criticised as paying insufficient attention to problems of power (e.g., Proctor, 2002; Smail, 2005). While such concepts as socioeconomic status, class, gender, sexual orientation, disability, race, ethnicity, and age all carry significant complexities of description and definition, they remain factors that can both influence access to psychotherapy and that also play a part in how the therapist and the client perceive each other in the consulting room (Rogers and Pilgrim, 2014; Pilgrim, 2020). We hold the position that as psychotherapists we need to remain curious about the person that walks into our consulting room, taking the trouble to explore that person's individual background and narratives, and understand their particular phenomenology. In this way, we can work within a richer frame of reference, appreciating, for example, important cultural differences or intergenerational complexities. A recent publication from the British Psychological Society has sought to revise the structural approach of current classifications with a narrative-based version of exploration. Johnstone et al. (2018), together with colleagues who have long been critical of formal classification systems and the objectification of presenting issues, propose a "Power, Threat, Meaning Framework" for the alternative exploration and understanding of a client's presenting issues (Johnstone et al., 2018). Instead of a focus on "symptoms", they propose an exploration with the client based on a series of questions such as "What has happened to you?", "How did it affect you?", "What sense did you make of it?", and "What did you have to do to survive?". This represents a crucial contextual location of the client's presenting issues, enabling the practitioner to formulate a contextual-based response in terms of "treatment". There is also the interesting interface between how the client and the therapist might answer these different questions!

In terms of a practice based response located in the arts, the client might draw a map of the journey that they and their families have travelled to the point of the client's birth, and possibly then a timeline that marks some of the main positive and challenging events that have shaped their own journey so far – a kind of visual autobiography. This could be something that could be explored in the moment and could also be returned to in future sessions. The activity might also reveal interesting differences between the therapist and the client that might have relevance to the therapeutic journey. Another approach would be for the client to draw an outline around their body, so that they could paint inside to share their feelings and the traces of any trauma, intergenerational trauma, and/ or oppression, supporting both the therapist and the client to take account of identity markers such as race, gender, or class.

The person-to-person relationship

The person-to-person relationship in psychotherapy has to do with the potential real here-and-now position of both the client and the therapist in the current time and the ways in which the therapist and the client meet each other in adopting such a stance. In this situation, the therapist and the client meet each other with an emphasis that is not on different roles, but on each as a human being. This creates a situation where each is potentially changed by the other. Spagnuolo Lobb, in the context of Gestalt psychotherapy, describes this as "a co-creation of a new contact boundary" (Spagnuolo Lobb, 2008, p. 123). Martin Buber distinguishes between an I–Thou and an I–It relationship, with the I-Thou highlighting a real or core meeting between persons (Buber, 1958). Hycner (1993) distinguishes between the "dialogical-interpersonal" and the "dialectic-intrapsychic" relationships within psychotherapy with the former focus highlighting the space between where "[I]t is the human spirit that permeates our every interaction" (Hycner and Jacobs, 1995, p. 3). Jacobs and Hycner (2008) go on to develop further these relational dialogic processes, highlighting their importance in the therapeutic setting. Daniel Stern also draws attention to the centrality of "the now moment" of meeting as a significant change moment in the process of psychotherapy and more broadly as a process that supports vitality and growth (Stern, 2004, 2010). These moments of real meeting are very likely to occur in the course of the different relationships that we have referred to earlier, for example, in sorting out the complexities of a co-constructed enactment. We consider that it is in the interest of psychotherapy effectiveness that the therapist is available for such meetings. We are also aware that such a focus can become more prominent towards the end of the therapeutic contract when the therapist and the client are reviewing their work together and preparing for an ending.

Although holding a position that is securely located in the current time zone can be challenging for both parties, there is the reality that clients do make a real-time commitment to make an appointment with a therapist, find a way to travel to this appointment, to manage the "therapeutic hour", and to return safely to their other worlds on departure from this experience. Also, psychotherapists, especially by the time that they are qualified, should have had extensive experience of their own psychotherapeutic issues in their personal therapy and the ways in which any of these might detract from a potential here-and-now interaction with a client. With regard to a "real" meeting, we also need to think about self-disclosure on the part of the therapist. There is a general feeling in the clinical and research literature on this issue that honesty is important and that, for example, if the therapist feels that they have made a mistake, they are willing to own up to this and to discuss the issue with the client. However, we believe that it is important that a practitioner thinks carefully about self-disclosure and considers the clinical implications of such interactions (Maroda, 2010; Yalom, 2002).

In drawing on the arts in exploring these issues, the psychotherapist might use the seven art forms to explore the resources available in therapy, getting to know these and what they might offer. They might help the client to notice how they feel as they hold, use it or experience the art form kinaesthetically, or explore these sensations and what they seem to express and compare them with other art forms, as they explore the therapy room. The use of the arts can also be used to share how the client has understood the feeling, relationship, or experience that they have brought to the therapist, letting them change or develop the image, so that it really captures their experience more fully. The client might also be encouraged to start keeping an art journal that could provide a supportive and containing space between their sessions. Images could then be brought back to therapy to help them to share their feelings and experiences.

Concluding Comments

We have attempted to illuminate what we think of as a number of complex and interesting ideas and practices in the context of integrative arts psychotherapy that we hope will be of value both to students and to more experienced practising therapists. These ideas are evolving as new research and innovative practices bring more nuances to light. In the last few decades, in particular, we have seen the emergence of many exciting new ideas, more recently highlighting the importance of implicit body processes and related ways in which both the therapist and the client are communicating with each other quite out of their individual awareness. The six relational frames that we outline seem to us to cover a number of key processes relevant to an understanding of what happens in psychotherapy, the potential for change in that setting, and the requirement for specific understandings and skills on the part of the therapist. While sometimes feeling daunted about how much there is to track, read, learn, and reflect on, occasionally brain-hurtlingly so, we remain energised and excited about these developments and what they can offer to the persons, lives, and contextual systems of our clients.

In the chapters that follow, you will see how different integrative arts psychotherapists have used this framework in a range of ways in their practice; how it enables them to develop a unique, creative, and holistic approach for an individual client or group that draws together a range of relevant theory and integrates the seven art forms. There will also be a focus on ways in which the psychotherapist can grade and pace their work in a collaborative way, as the journey unfolds.

References

Beebe, B. & Lachmann, F. M. (2014) *The Origins of Attachment: Infant Research and Adult Treatment*. New York and London: Routledge.

Bordin, E. S. (1994) Theory and Research on the Therapeutic Working Alliance: New Directions. In Horvath, A. O. & Greenberg, L. S. (Eds.) *The Working Alliance: Theory, Research and Practice*. New York: Wiley.

Bromberg, P. M. (2011) *The Shadow of the Tsunami and the Growth of the Relational Mind*. New York and London: Routledge.

Buber, M. (1958) *I and Thou*. Translated by R. G. Smith (2nd edition). Edinburgh: T & T Clark.

Clarkson, P. (1990) A Multiplicity of Psychotherapeutic Relationships. *British Journal of Psychotherapy*, 7(2), pp. 148–163.

Clarkson, P. (1995) *The Therapeutic Relationship*. London: Whurr.

Cozolino, L. (2017) *The Neuroscience of Psychotherapy: Healing the Social Brain* (3rd edition). London: W. W. Norton & Co.

Dana, D. (2020) *Polyvagal Exercises for Safety and Connection.* New York: W. W. Norton & Co.

DeYoung, P. A. (2015) *Relational Psychotherapy: A Primer.* New York: Routledge.

Diagnostic and Statistical Manual of Mental Disorders (2013) (DSM-5, 5th edition). Washington, DC: American Psychiatric Publishing.

Epstein, M. (1995) *Psychotherapy from a Buddhist Perspective: Thoughts Without a Thinker.* New York: Basic Books.

Ferenczi, S. (1994) *Final Contributions to the Problems and Methods of Psycho-Analysis.* Edited by Michael Balint. Translated by Eric Mosbacher and others. London: Karnac.

Fisher, J. (2017) *Healing the Fragmented Selves of Trauma Survivors.* New York and London: Routledge.

Freud, S. (1913) On the Beginning of Treatment: Further Recommendations on the Technique of Psychoanalysis. In Strachey, J. (Ed.) *Standard Edition of the Complete Psychological Works of Sigmund Freud* (Vol. 12). London: Hogarth.

Freud, S. (1913/1940) The Technique of Psychoanalysis. In Strachey, J. (Ed.) *Standard Edition of the Complete Psychological Works of Sigmund Freud* (Vol. 23). London: Hogarth.

Gergen, K. J. (2009) *An Invitation to Social Construction* (2nd edition). London: Sage.

Gilbert, M. & Orlans, V. (2011) *Integrative Therapy: 100 Key Points and Techniques.* London: Routledge.

Gilbert, P. (2018) *Living Like Crazy* (2nd edition). York: Annwyn House.

Gilbert, P. & Choden (2013) *Mindful Compassion.* London: Constable and Robinson Ltd.

Hagman, G., Paul, H. & Zimmermann, P. B. (Eds.) (2019) *Intersubjective Self Psychology.* London and New York: Routledge.

Heimann, P. (1950) On Countertransference. *International Journal of Psychoanalysis, 31,* pp. 31–34.

Horvath, A. O., Del Re, A. C., Flückiger, C. & Symonds, D. (2011) Alliance in Individual Psychotherapy. In Norcross, J. C. (Ed.) *Psychotherapy Relationship That Work: Evidence-Based Responsiveness* (2nd edition). New York: Oxford University Press.

Hycner, R. (1993) *Between Person and Person.* New York: The Gestalt Journal Press.

Hycner, R. & Jacobs, L. (1995) *The Healing Relationship in Gestalt Therapy.* New York: The Gestalt Journal Press.

International Classification of Diseases (2021) (ICD11, 11th revision). Geneva: World Health Organization.

Jacobs, L. & Hycner, R. (Eds.) (2008) *Relational Approaches in Gestalt Therapy.* New York: Routledge, Taylor & Francis Group.

Johnstone, L., Boyle, M., Cromby, J., Dillon, J., Harper, D., Kinderman, P., Longden, E., Pilgrim, D. & Read, J. (2018). *The Power Threat Meaning Framework: Towards the Identification of Patterns in Emotional Distress, Unusual Experiences and Troubled or Troubling Behaviour, as an Alternative to Functional Psychiatric Diagnosis.* Leicester: British Psychological Society.

Jung, C. G. (1959–1969) The Archetypes and the Collective Unconscious. In Read, M., Fordham, M., Adler, G., McGuire, W. (Eds.) & Hull, R. F. C. (Trans.) *The Collected Works of C. G. Jung.* Bollingham Series (2nd edition, Vol. 9, p. 1). London: Princeton University Press.

Knox, J. (2003) *Archetype, Attachment, Analysis: Jungian Psychology and the-Emergent Mind.* London: Routledge.

Kohut, H. (1984) *How Does Analysis Cure?* Chicago: The University of Chicago Press.

Lapworth, P. & Sills, C. (2010) *Integration in Counselling & Psychotherapy: A Personal Approach* (2nd edition). London: Sage.

Maroda, K. J. (2010) *Psychodynamic Techniques: Working with Emotion in the Therapeutic Relationship.* New York: The Guilford Press.

McNamee, S. & Gergen, K. J. (Eds.) (1992) *Therapy as Social Construction.* London: Sage.

Norcross, J. C. (2010) The Therapeutic Relationship. In Duncan, B. L., Miller, S. D., Wampold, B. E. & Hubble, M. A. (Eds.) *The Heart and Soul of Change* (2nd edition). Washington, DC: American Psychological Association.

Norcross, J. C. & Goldfried, M. R. (Eds.) (2019) *Handbook of Psychotherapy Integration* (3rd edition). New York: Oxford University Press.

Norcross, J. C. & Lambert, M. J. (2011) Evidence-Based Therapy Relationships. In Norcross, J. C. (Ed.) *Psychotherapy Relationship That Work: Evidence-Based Responsiveness* (2nd edition). New York: Oxford University Press.

Orange, D. M., Atwood, G. E., & Stolorow, R. D. (1997) *Working Intersubjectively: Contextualism in Psychoanalytic Practice.* New York: Routledge.

Orlans, V. & Van Scoyoc, S. (2009) *A Short Introduction to Counselling Psychology.* London: Sage.

Papadopoulos, R. K. (Ed.) (2006) *The Handbook of Jungian Psychology: Theory, Practice and Applications.* London: Routledge.

Pilgrim, D. (2020) *Key Concepts in Mental Health* (5th edition). London: Sage.

Polster, E. (1995) *A Population of Selves: A Therapeutic Exploration of Personal Diversity.* San Francisco: Jossey-Bass.

Porges, S. W. & Dana, D. (Eds.) (2018) *Clinical Applications of The Polyvagal Theory.* New York: W. W. Norton & Co.

Proctor, G. (2002) *The Dynamics of Power in Counselling and Psychotherapy: Ethics, Politics and Practice.* Ross-on-Wye: PCCS Books.

Racker, H. (1968) *Transference and Countertransference.* London: Karnac.

Rogers, A. & Pilgrim, D. (2014) *A Sociology of Mental Health and Illness* (5th edition). Maidenhead: McGraw-Hill Education, Open University Press.

Rogers, C. R. (1959) A Theory of Therapy, Personality and Interpersonal Relationships, as Developed in the Client-Centered Framework. In Koch, S. (Ed.) *Psychology: A Study of Science, Vol. III. Formulations of the Person and the Social Context.* New York: McGraw-Hill.

Rogers, C. R. (1980) *A Way of Being.* Boston: Houghton Mifflin Company

Rowan, J. (2005) *The Transpersonal: Spirituality in Psychotherapy and Counselling* (2nd edition). London: Routledge.

Rycroft, C. (1979) *A Critical Dictionary of Psychoanalysis.* London: Penguin.

Safran, J. D. & Muran, J. C. (2006) Has the Concept of the Therapeutic Alliance Outlined its Usefulness? *Psychotherapy: Theory, Research, Practice, Training, 43*(3), pp. 286–291.

Sandler, J., Dare, C. & Holder, A. (1992) *The Patient and the Analyst.* London: Karnac.

Schore, A. N. (2019) *Right Brain Psychotherapy.* New York: W. W. Norton & Co.

Smail, D. (2005) *Power, Interest and Psychology: Elements of a Social Materialist Understanding of Distress.* Ross-on-Wye: PCCS Books.

Spagnuolo Lobb, M. (2008) The Therapeutic Relationship in Gestalt Therapy. In Jacobs, L. & Hycner, R. (Eds.) *Relational Approaches in Gestalt Therapy.* New York: Routledge, Taylor & Francis Group.

Sroufe, L. A., Egeland, B., Carlson, E. A. & Collins, W. A. (2005) *The Development of the Person: The Minnesota Study of Risk and Adaptation from Birth to Adulthood*. New York: The Guilford Press.

Steele, K., Boon, S. & van der Hart, O. (2017) *Treating Trauma-Related Dissociation: A Practical Integrative Approach*. New York: W. W. Norton & Co.

Stern, D. (2003) *The Interpersonal World of the Infant: A View from Psychoanalysis and Developmental Psychology* (2nd edition). London: Karnac (first published in 1985 by Basic Books).

Stern, D. N. (2004) *The Present Moment in Psychotherapy and Everyday Life*. New York: W. W. Norton & Company, Inc.

Stern, D. N. (2010) *Forms of Vitality: Exploring Dynamic Experience in Psychology, the Arts, Psychotherapy, and Development*. Oxford: Oxford University Press.

van der Kolk, B. (2014) *The Body Keeps the Score*. London: Allen Lane/Penguin.

West, W. (2000) *Psychotherapy and Spirituality*. London: Sage.

Yalom, I. D. (2002) *The Gift of Therapy*. London: Piatkus.

Part III

Creative integration in practice – working with individuals

Chapter 5

Hide and seek

Using the arts and the body to assist discovery and self-awareness

Tsafi Lederman

Introduction

For some psychotherapy clients, there is a delicate balance between being seen and being exposed. Winnicott (1965b) observed: "It is a sophisticated game of hide-and-seek, in which it is a joy to be hidden and disaster not to be found". Using the arts and focusing on the body in psychotherapy can support the process of discovery and awareness within the co-created relational field between the therapist and the client (Perls, 1992; Francesetti, 2015). The focus will be on developing insight and potential for change through attending to verbal and non-verbal communication, metaphors, emerging images, and the interchange between embodiment and externalisation to enable this process.

Hide and seek is a process full of dilemmas. Clients engage in the therapeutic encounter hope to improve aspects of their life and explore what really matters and what gives meaning to their current situation (seek). From the first contact, the exploration of the present and planning for the future are coloured by past experiences and relationships. They want to talk about what troubles them, but they don't know if they can trust, disclose, and expose difficult aspects of their life (hide). The co-created therapeutic relationship provides the essential container that holds the client's material (Anderson, 1992).

The longing to be found and seen can be impeded by the fear of being "found out" and exposed. There might be a fear of re-experiencing trauma, overwhelming emotions, issues of shame, and ambivalence around the consequence of becoming more aware. Additionally, fear of being criticised, perhaps a legacy from an earlier experience of impingement prejudice or disadvantage, may have led to withdrawal into a "quiet isolation" (Winnicott, 1988). These feelings may be hidden from self and the caregiver, or a response to living in a social system in which they experience others' prejudices. Kalsched (1996) describes the hide process as a self-care system designed to protect the individual; potentially, cutting off attachment and suppressing the possibilities of true-self living. There may also be loyalty to historical or cultural messages about secrecy – that "dirty washing" should not be done in public.

Clients can also be hidden in therapy because they can't access a clear sense of an issue. Bollas (1987) refers to this as the "Unthought Known"; what we may

DOI: 10.4324/9781003155676-9

"know" but are unable to think about or discuss. The use of creative modalities within the safety of the therapeutic space allows unconscious material to emerge, providing a space for clients who may, otherwise, find it difficult to engage with their hide and seek patterns.

Implications and applications

Using visual and embodied art forms can enable access and exploration of layers of meanings. By engaging with different art forms, we experience sensations and access an implicit "non-conscious" knowledge – the "implicit knowing" that lies beyond thinking (Banella et al., 2018). It is within the spectrum of "seeking to be found" that the client can discover and reveal what has been concealed or lost in the contact with self and others and the words to articulate this.

In my work as a body psychotherapist, Gestalt and Integrative Arts Psychotherapist, I use two main pathways to explore the implicit knowledge, focusing on body processes and exploring emerging images and metaphors. This approach can expand the possibilities for expression and self-care. This way of working has been informed by an integration of Object Relations, Gestalt, TA, Intersubjectivity, Humanistic phenomenology, and the arts within the Therapeutic Relational Model (Gilbert & Orlans, 2011; Clarkson, 2003). Based on the six facets of the therapeutic relationship, the therapist's "way of being" in the intersubjective field changes according to the client's process and needs.

Intention and intervention form and are informed by the therapist moving between different therapeutic stances, positioning themselves as "object, self-object, and as subject" (Stark, 2000). The transition between the different intentions can be complex, involving conscious and unconscious processes that can lead to misattunement. Awareness of the therapeutic relationship being a body/mind contract within an embodied matrix can support attunement and movement within the six-relationship framework and between the different art forms.

Verbal and non-verbal communication

The shift from drive theory to object relations theory emphasises the importance of the embodied relational field. Winnicott (1987, p. 88) stated that "[t]here is no such a thing as a baby without the mother", reinforced by "there is no body without another body" (Orbach, 2003, p. 11). The self is shaped through the interpersonal relationship. Merleau-Ponty suggests that consciousness is always embodied consciousness as it is experienced through the body (Merleau-Ponty, 1968; Jones, 2007). Paying attention to the two bodies in the therapeutic exchange, in individual psychotherapy, includes an understanding that all our experiences exist within the context of all our previous life/cultural interactions – a constant dialogue between the two bodies.

How the therapist listens and responds to the client's body, within the "talking cure", plays an important part in creating trust and open communication. Schore

(2009) describes this process as "a shift from the explicit, verbal, rational domain to the implicit, integrative, non-verbal, bodily based emotional domain". Inviting clients to reflect on the "felt sense" of their experience can help the integration of subjective knowledge (Gendlin, 1979). Attending to the language of the body includes attention to posture, eye contact, breathing, tone of voice, gestures, movement, energy, and levels of vitality (Boadella, 1987; Stern, 2010). It is followed by somatic inquiry and tracking the phenomenological process. This can reveal the gap and conflict between the client's words and the unspoken story held in their body; for example, a client who talks about a new relationship being "perfect" while her hand gesture is pushing something away from her body. Phenomenological inquiry into the meaning of this gesture, focusing on the movement without words, revealed fear and ambivalence about the new "perfect" relationship. Attention to the whole person, words and body, can expand our understanding of the range of emotions that are not in awareness.

The rich possibilities of working with a range of art forms invite the client to externalise and project onto an image and objects including expression through embodiment. Alternating between the projected and embodied process, attending to and tracking the client's process, can support connection with unknown material and help the client's split-off parts to emerge and to be owned (Osherson & Krugman, 1990).

Skaife (2001) highlights the link between spoken and visual language. Early language is based on the senses and expressed through painting, sculpture, performance, and poetry. Therefore, gestures are not separated from thought and language is a gesture (Heidegger, 1968). Observation of the client's embodied phenomenology while creating an art image is as important as what is being created. Spontaneous gesture is "the true self in action" (Winnicott, 1965a, p. 148). Painting or movement can be seen as an extension of a gesture into an artistic form.

Attunement

Beyond words, the therapist's own body awareness enhances their attuned communication to the client's non-verbal expressions (Aitken & Trevarthen, 1997). This attunement is similar to the mother–baby communication by observing, sensing, and responding. Similarly, the therapist can develop an embodied presence in response to the client's changing "vitality affect" (Stern, 1985). This creates a form of "listening with the body"; an attunement to self and other that enables embodied presence and dialogue. Stern (1985) describes this as "affect attunement". Through somatic intersubjectivity, the embodied presence of the therapist supports the client's ability to express themselves as they feel more met and understood.

Embodied attunement to the client enables a deeper connection with the implicit, hidden aspects of their distress. Aitken and Trevarthen (1997) describes attunement as being felt and seen by another, to which we can add "being found by another", and can be supported by the therapist's empathy. Attunement can inform empathy but is different from it by being a moment-to-moment interaction. This process can be enhanced by the use of the arts and is a bidirectional process where the arts can inform the body and where the body can inform the arts (see the case study). Within this process, the client is invited to reflect and find meaning in the emerging themes, images, and narratives.

Tracking the non-verbal expression, following the impulse and dynamics of the physical expression, allows the body to tell a story that is held in the internal embodied construct.

Metaphors and the embodied metaphor

Images and metaphors can access implicit embodied knowledge. Burns (2007) points out that metaphors can convey much with few words, are evocative, and easily remembered. Sunderland (2000) suggests that the mind chooses images and metaphor as ways of processing powerful feelings in our past or present, as well as fears and hopes for the future. Metaphors have a powerful connection with the unconscious and can offer safety for clients to go beyond habitual inhibitions, enabling mobilisation and release of affect (Siegelman, 1990; Mackewn, 1997).

Embodiment of the client's metaphors is referred to here as "Embodied Metaphor Process" (a variation of this approach is also used in bodywork, movement, and drama therapy). The embodied metaphor can develop from verbal and non-verbal expression, through a physical exploration of the metaphor's content. It can also be an embodied response to any image, painting, sculpture, or an object in the sandtray. For example, a vulnerable client painted an image of an oak tree and was invited to "become the tree". Speaking in the first person from their embodied experience, they stated that they felt strong, more centred, and grounded. Similarly, the common metaphor "I carry the world on my shoulders" can communicate an embodied experience and be personalised by exploring it through embodiment. A meaningful narrative can emerge using phenomenological inquiry. It can support a conversation about the experience beyond a figure of speech. Additionally, the embodied metaphor can develop into expression through an embodied stance or movement. This is somewhat different from Schaverien's (1992) embodied image in which the image itself can communicate strongly without having to physically engage the body in action.

Embodiment of image and metaphor can be used with clients who find it difficult to connect to their somatic experience. In this phenomenological exploration, a link is made between language and the sensations that arise from the body. Communication through metaphors creates a shared language between the therapist and the client and may help open up difficult conversations. Staying with the metaphor can provide safety by both concealing and revealing, which can enhance the client's self-awareness and experience of being understood, i.e., being "found" and "seen".

Awareness can have two forms: conceptual and embodied (Fogel, 2013). Conceptual awareness is the insight and understanding that is acquired over time and can be habitual in nature. Embodied awareness is the experience based on the sensations arising from the body in conjunction with emotions, memories, impulses, and images (Gendlin, 1979). A therapeutic relationship that flows between the two forms of awareness creating an embodied somatic connection between the client and the therapist can support the potential for discovery, change, and a shift in perception from self-knowledge to an embodied self-awareness.

Projections and externalising

Using the arts, metaphors, and images can be externalised and projected into a physical form through creative expression. The clients can use a blank piece of paper or the sandtray as a contained space to "hold" objects that symbolise their inner world.

Within this space, they can experiment with creating images and narratives that explore new possibilities. They can also become familiar with the parts of themselves that have been hidden or placed in others. Here, the more hidden aspects of themselves can emerge, giving voice to internal conflicts and offering a safe place to experiment with new possibilities. This offers the client a way to become aware and take back their projections of unwanted thoughts and emotions that have, historically, been rejected. Hidden abilities and qualities can then come to light, be owned, and help integrate a new internal relationship.

Externalising offers an overview and distancing, yet paradoxically, it can bring us closer to ourselves (Jennings, 1992). Externalising and images offer the client a relationship with the problem rather than identifying with it as a dominant aspect of themselves. This enables reflection and creation of a new narrative to understand and manage it in a more resourced and skilful way (White, 1990). For example, the part of self that is highly critical may be seen as an unwanted visitor; an inner critic that stops and spoils any creative attempt. Distinguishing the inner critic as a separated part of self can help attenuate its power.

Landscapes of selves and stories we tell ourselves

Externalising and projection onto an art form may involve a creation of a landscape, images of place, self, and the self within its environment (landscape of selves). This enables a tangible connection with unknown, forgotten, and neglected parts mentioned previously. The image provides an integrative overview of the relationships between the different aspects of the self and the environment. The reflection can include an exploration of intrapsychic, interpsychic, and intersubjective processes. Through reflection on these landscapes, personal stories, including the stories we tell ourselves, may emerge and play a vital role in understanding limiting or supporting beliefs that impact our attitudes and behaviour. These internal narratives can be explored through the arts to re-evaluate their meaning in relation to the past, present, and possible futures.

Sharing stories through the arts can shine light on introjects and script messages that inform a unique organisation of self. These not only impact our beliefs and behaviour but will also manifest in the way we carry the embodied narrative of our life – the way we walk, talk, breathe, hold ourselves, and our contact with the environment, referred to here as "somatic organisation". Organisation of the self in its environment is an attempt to adapt and stay regulated and is part of our creative adjustment (Perls et al., 1951).

An exploration of links between the image, emerging narrative, and how they manifest in the body can bring about a new relational stance, posture, and movement behaviour to redefine current personal values and authentic, true self-expression.

Case example

This case example runs over several sessions and illustrates integrated practice involving embodied approaches and the arts when working with the process of hide and seek. (The case material was discussed with the client, anonymised, and presented with her consent.) The client is a 40-year-old mother of two who was trying to develop her career after a break. A good working alliance has been established, and person-to-person, reparative, and transferential relational experiences emerged throughout the therapeutic process.

In one particular session, the client arrived in a low mood, unsure of the cause, and without a clear understanding or insight into her feelings. As she talked about her mood, I asked her what she was experiencing in her body. She was aware of tension in her right shoulder. Using phenomenological tracking and attuning to her embodied awareness, I asked her to stay with the tension and see what it felt like. At that point, there was a tiny movement in her right shoulder which brought to her awareness of the need to move. As she was moving her shoulder, I tracked the expression on her body and asked "Is there anything it wants to do?". An impulse to move emerged starting at her elbow, followed by her hand, and eventually involved her whole arm. As she moved her arm up and down, she said that it felt as if she had a wing.

Tracking the embodied image and movement, I encouraged the wing's movement to develop and expand. As the movement developed, I noticed a change in her facial expression. After a further enquiry into what was happening with the rest of her body, the client noticed the left side of her body felt frozen and that she felt sad. She said, "It's as if I have only one wing". I asked her to notice what was happening in her still left arm. She said:

> It's frozen, it's frozen with fear, it can't move, I can only have one wing. I can't fly, I can't get this project off the ground; It's often like this when I am trying to engage with any new projects – I get stuck.

The metaphor of having one wing while the other was frozen highlighted a habitual pattern that had stopped her from following opportunities in the past. In order to bring both parts of her body into relationship, I invited identification through a dialogue between the "wings", addressing the dilemma arising between the still wing and the moving wing.

Staying with image and metaphor that emerged through the gestalt experiment (Zinker, 1977) and phenomenological tracking, followed by her embodied dialogue, the client became more aware of her habitual pattern of "hiding" both in her conflict about new projects and in other contexts.

Subsequent session

A subsequent session took us further in our understanding of the history behind this conflict. It began when the client noticed a tube of pink paint (in my art collection), which she wanted to explore. She started to make marks on the paper, which eventually formed pink brush strokes jutting out from a half-circle shape. Looking excited and playful in her movements while painting, she commented; "It looks like a tutu". This evoked memories of excitement at receiving her first tutu when she was 3 years old. Whilst observing the image and tracking her physical expression, there was a shift in her affect. Dialogical inquiry led to a further elaboration of this childhood memory. She added, "I remember when I got my first tutu, I was so excited. I put it on and danced on the coffee table. My parents got very angry and told to me, stop showing off and get off the table immediately". At that moment, I noticed her body contracting and inquired about this experience. The client talked about feeling smaller, wishing to disappear, while looking down, curling her body, and bringing her arms together. The wish to diminish and hide made me think about the embodied expression of shame (Van der Kolk, 2014; Mollon, 2002). The client remembered the shame and shock of those moments, moving between being very excited to feeling that she has done something wrong. She remembered the voice and the expression on her mother's face – the look of disapproval and disappointment. This experience was internalised as an introject of being "bad and wrong". Observing and listening, I was aware of the impact of the client's process on my body. Empathically attuning, I felt my body getting tense, I was holding my breath, I noticed how angry I felt on behalf of the "little girl". I invited the client to stay in contact with me by responding to her distress and validating her experience.

Recollecting the impact of her parent's disapproval, noticing her embodied experience, she said, "I will never speak to my child like this". I asked her to think about what she might have said to one of her daughters in a similar situation. We stood up and moved away from the picture. I enquired about her somatic experience. She imagined the tone of voice, facial expression, and the words that she could use when speaking to her daughter. With warmth, she acknowledged the excitement and beauty of her dance as a child. She pointed out that the coffee table may not be strong enough to stand on and, perhaps they could create a space on the floor that would be the "stage". I invited her to imagine how this response could have been addressed to her younger self, she moved to a different area of the room and imagined it as a stage. She remembered the girl with the tutu, taking in the accepting supportive voice, letting the voice inform sensations, and letting her body follow her impulse for expression. This led her to move her body in a new dance of "pride". From this embodied experience of free expression, I invited a phenomenological inquiry into the newly formed somatic organisation, observing the shift from shame to pride in her movements and posture. Healthy pride can be understood as the opposite polarity of the contracted shame stance (Sanderson, 2015).

Staying open and curious about the emerging sensations, images, metaphors, and gestures enabled the client to speak about the experience of being "frozen" and "wanting to disappear" (hiding). My presence, being grounded and open to notice sensations, impulses including images and feelings, created an embodied field that supported the client's spontaneous expression (Mitchelle, 2000; Kepner, 2003; Totton, 2018). Winnicott (1971) suggested that the psyche needs to be rooted in the soma in order for spontaneous gestures to emerge. An inhibition of the spontaneous gesture is related to the false self, whereas creativity and play can support a sense of true self.

The image of the girl with the tutu became a shared figure of speech over time and as a metaphor for the "hide" pattern. This image appeared and disappeared in relation to her patterns of contact and withdrawal. In a subsequent session, a further link was made between the somatic unconscious expression and a three-dimensional visual representation of her inner conflict. This process was exter-nalised in the sandtray as a small girl with a tutu facing a giant green monster (Figure 5.1). The girl was trying to turn her body away "looking anxious". Over

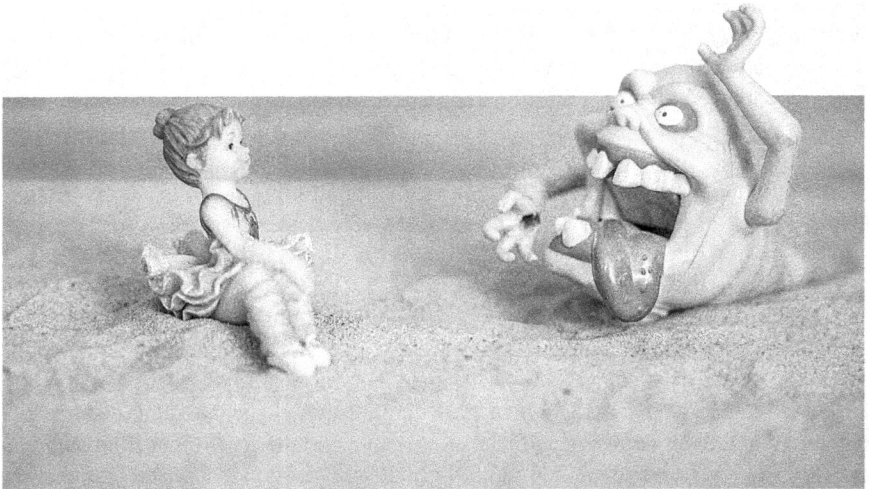

Figure 5.1 The girl with the pink dress and the inner critic

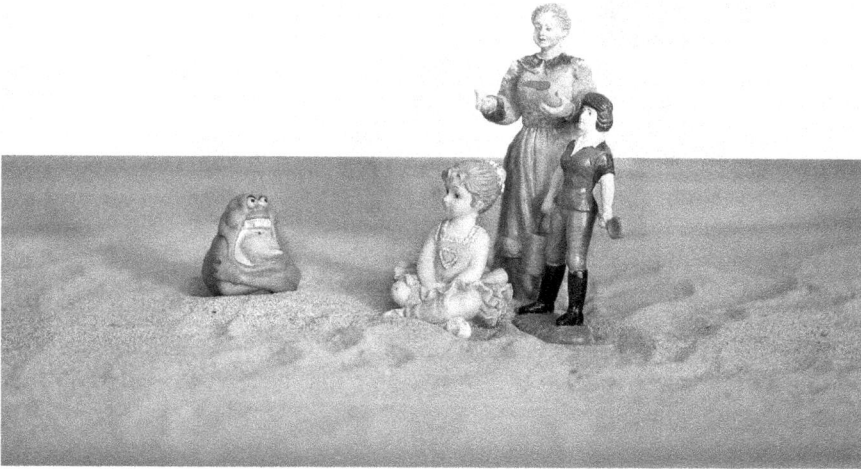

Figure 5.2 The girl with the pink dress: developing self-support over time

time, this developed into another scene where the girl was facing a smaller green monster; accompanied by a young woman who she described as a hard-working farm lady and another figure of a maternal woman with open arms (Figure 5.2).

The green monster represented her introjected inner critic. In the second image, the smaller monster represented her progress where the inner critic was less dominant. The green monster has been cut down to size and was no longer a threat to her authentic female strength. The adult female figures in the image represented her adult and nurturing parent ego states who could now stand by her, enabling access to these qualities (Berne et al., 1973).

The externalised exploration helped reflect on her process of change. The client's image and embodied knowledge of the hide and seek patterns had become a resource that supported her empowerment, self-regulation, and choice. Through her body awareness and finding an image and metaphor for it, she was able to recognise her different contextual ego states and use her awareness for self-care; as Perls (1978) observed, therapy can help the clients develop their own support for desired contact or withdrawal.

Embodied script

The client's embodied experience of her introjects from her family and culture became part of a "life script" (Berne et al., 1973; Baumgardner & Perls, 1975). She internalised the message of "don't show off" as the acceptable way to be. This led to a pattern of withdrawing and hiding her talent and capabilities, an embodied script that shaped her way of being in the world. There was a habitual somatic pattern of muscle tension, which could be triggered at a time of stress (Reich, 1980). This protective mechanism was an attempt to avoid an experience of shame and humiliation. It formed an "embodied script" – a habitual, personal somatic organisation in posture, movement, muscle tension, breathing patterns, as well as the impulse to move (seek) or withdraw (hide).

The embodied script became evident and exaggerated when the client recalled her childhood experience with the tutu. This brought up strong feelings of shame reflecting in the wish to hide. This was experienced at the time as a lonely place for her. I was reminded, here, of Wheeler's (1995) emphasis not to try to "remove shame" but to support the new and different experience of shame by being connected, rather than isolated. The awareness of her self-protective strategies (need to hide) was met by the acknowledgment and validation of her experience. This enabled her to find a language to describe her "isolated sad place". This led to a shift from a retroflected anger to finding an authentic adult voice.

Enabling presence

Throughout the work, my own body awareness informed my therapeutic presence and interventions, noticing her contraction, change in breathing, and the impulse to protect the girl with the pink tutu. I wanted to validate and respond to the child's creative and playful expression in a way that would enable a different experience of self – a reparative relationship (Clarkson, 2003). Noticing my body process in relation to the girl's "shrinking body" brought awareness of the developmental needs of the client for acceptance, validation, and being seen and not being an "impingement" (Winnicott, 1958).

Playing with the pink paint, within the safe "holding" and "facilitating environment" allowed a greater depth and reflection (Winnicott, 1962). A story emerged from the body process and from the painting in which, paradoxically, attunement to the non-verbal process of the art making allowed the art image to emerge and form a verbal narrative. McNiff (2004) suggested that "Images generate stories, imaginal dialogue . . . they also act directly on our bodies, minds and senses". Within the therapeutic relationship, the implicit relational exchange informed my somatic counter-transference. I was aware of an impulse to support the girl, which at times I held back. This provided a space for her adult ego state to emerge, enabling a shift from the reparative transferential to a "real relationship" exchange.

Conclusion

This chapter explored the hide and seek process in therapy. It demonstrates how the use of the body and the arts can expand communication awareness and potential for insights and change. The knowledge and awareness from the image and body can help the client develop resourcefulness for self-regulation.

Within the hide and seek patterns, there is a flow between what is known and unknown, visible and invisible within the therapeutic relationship. This polarity can be understood as a continuum in which new awareness and choice can emerge.

The client's use and experience of her body and the arts enabled a deeper contact with her embodied sense of self. The creative expression could then emerge and be recognised by the embodied therapist, supporting the client's process of change and true self-experience.

Using different art modalities can enable a flow between embodiment and externalisation supporting the emerging narrative. Within the context of a safe environment, an attuned response to this narrative can provide the client with a deeper understanding of their hide and seek patterns, out of which growth and development can take place.

References

Aitken, K.J. and Trevarthen, C. (1997) Self/other organization in human psychological development. *Development and Psychopathology*, 9(4), pp. 653–677.

Anderson, R. ed. (1992) *Clinical lectures on Klein and Bion* (No. 14). London: Psychology Press.

Banella, F.E., Speranza, A.M. and Tronick, E. (2018) Mutual regulation and unique forms of implicit relational knowing. *Rassegna di Psicologia*, 35(3), pp. 67–76.

Baumgardner, P. and Perls, F. (1975) *Legacy from Fritz*. Palo Alto, CA: Science and Behavior Books.

Berne, E., Steiner, C. and Dusay, J. (1973) Transactional analysis. *Direct Psychotherapy*, 1.

Boadella, D. (1987) *Lifestreams: An introduction to biosynthesis*. London: Routledge and Kegan Paul.

Bollas, C. (1987) *The shadow of the object*. Abingdon: Routledge.

Burns, G.W. ed. (2007) *Healing with stories: Your casebook collection for using therapeutic metaphors*. New York: John Wiley & Sons.

Clarkson, P. (2003) *The therapeutic relationship*. New York: John Wiley & Sons.

Fogel, A. (2013) *Body sense; the science and practice of emotional self-awareness*. New York: Norton.

Francesetti, G. (2015) From individual symptoms to psychopathological fields. Towards a field perspective on clinical human suffering. *British Gestalt Journal*, 24, pp. 5–19.

Gendlin, E. (1979) *Focusing*. London: Bantan Books.

Gilbert, M. and Orlans, V. (2011) *Integrative therapy. 100 key points and techniques*. London: Routledge.

Heidegger, M. and Gray, J.G. (1968) *What is called thinking*. London: Harperstock Books.

Jennings, S. (1992) *Dramatherapy with families, groups and individuals: Waiting in the wings*. London: Jessica Kingsley Publishers.

Jones, P. (2007) *Drama as therapy volume 1: Theory, practice and research*. Abingdon: Routledge.

Kalsched, D. (1996) *The inner world of trauma: Archetypal defences of the personal spirit*. Abingdon: Routledge.

Kepner, J. (2003) The embodied field. *British Gestalt Journal*, 12(1), pp. 6–14.

Mackewn, J. (1997) *Developing gestalt counselling*. London: Sage.

McNiff, S. (2004) *Art heals: How creativity cures the soul*. Boston: Shambhala.

Merleau-Ponty, M. (1968) *The primacy of perception and other essays*. Evanstone, IL: Northwester University Press.

Mitchelle, S.A. (2000) *Relationality: From attachment to intersubjectivity*. London: The Analytic Press.

Mollon, P. (2002) *Shame and jealousy: The hidden turmoils*. Abingdon: Routledge.

Orbach, S. (2003) Part I: There is no such thing as a body. *British Journal of Psychotherapy*, 20(1), pp. 3–16.

Osherson, S. and Krugman, S. (1990) Men, shame, and psychotherapy. *Psychotherapy: Theory, Research, Practice, Training*, 27(3), p. 327.

Perls, F.S. (1978) Finding the self through gestalt therapy. *Gestalt Journal*, 1(1), Winter.

Perls, F.S., Hefferline, R. and Goodman, P. (1951/1994) *Gestalt therapy: Excitement & growth in the human personality*. New York: The Gestalt Journal Press.

Perls, L. (1992) *Living at the boundary*. Maine: Gestalt Journal Press.

Reich, W. (1980) *Character analysis*. London: Macmillan.

Sanderson, C. (2015) *Counselling skills for working with shame*. London: Jessica Kingsley Publishers.

Schaverien, J. (1992) *The revealing image: Analytical art psychotherapy in theory and practice*. London: Tavistock/Routledge.

Schore, A.N. (2009) Relational trauma and the developing right brain: An interface of psychoanalytic self psychology and neuroscience. *Self and Systems*, 1159, pp. 189–203.

Siegelman, E.Y. (1990) *Metaphor and meaning in psychotherapy*. New York and London: Guilford Press.

Skaife, S. (2001) Making visible: Art therapy and intersubjectivity. *International Journal of Art Therapy: Inscape*, 6(2), pp. 40–50.

Stark, M. (2000) *Modes of therapeutic action*. New York: Rowman & Littlefield.

Stern, D.N. (1985) *The inter personal world of the infant*. New York: Basic Books.

Stern, D.N. (2010) *Forms of vitality; Exploration dynamic experience in psychology. The arts, psychotherapy, and development*. Oxford: Oxford University Press.

Sunderland, M. (2000) *Using story telling as a therapeutic tool with children*. London: Taylor & Francis Group.

Totton, N. (2018) *Embodied relating: The ground of psychotherapy*. Abingdon: Routledge.

Van der Kolk, B. (2014) *The body keeps the score: Mind, brain and body in the transformation of trauma*. London: Penguin.

Wheeler, G. (1995) Shame in two paradigms of therapy. *The British Gestalt Journal*, 4(2).

White, M. and Epston, D. (1990) *Narrative means to therapeutic ends*. New York: W. W. Norton.

Winnicott, D.W. (1958) The capacity to be alone. *International Journal of Psycho-Analysis*, 39, pp. 416–420.

Winnicott, D.W. (1962) The aims of psycho-analytical treatment (pp. 166–170). In *The maturational processes and the facilitating environment*. New York: Basic Books.

Winnicott, D.W. (1965a) Ego distortion in terms of true and false self (pp. 140–152). In *The maturational process and the facilitating environment: Studies in the theory of emotional development*. New York: International University Press Inc.

Winnicott, D.W. (1965b) The maturational processes and the facilitating environment (p. 186). In *Studies in the theory of emotional development*. London, New York: Karnac.

Winnicott, D.W. (1971) *Playing and reality*. London and New York: Routledge.
Winnicott, D.W. (1987) *The child, the family, and the outside world*. Cambridge, MA: Perseus.
Winnicott, D.W. (1988) *Human nature*. New York: Schocken Books.
Zinker, J. (1977) *Creative process in gestalt therapy*. New York: Vintage Books.

Chapter 6

Embodying metaphor

Visual art, movement, and the body

Gary Nash

Introduction

The aim of this chapter is to describe my approach when working collaboratively with clients to facilitate a movement of creative energy that is initiated, developed, and completed through the creative cycle. I will describe facilitating this movement by highlighting the use of the body, the visual arts, and metaphor within the person-to-person relationship (Clarkson, 1989; Gilbert & Orlans, 2011) and from a "dialogic" stance (Mackewn, 1997; Mann, 2010). This work can emerge and be explored most effectively in therapeutic relationships when there is a working alliance in place and the client is able and willing to engage collaboratively in the creative and metaphoric forms of expressive arts in psychotherapy.

The use of visual arts media, metaphor, and the expressive experience of the body is the focus of this chapter, ending with reference to the use of the "retrospective review" (Schaverien, 1993). The case vignettes are from my work with adults in private practice; pseudonyms are used to protect identity. The vignettes are written with full involvement and consent, with permission to use the images given.

Art, psychotherapy, and cycles of creativity

A creative experience in psychotherapy involves preparation, engagement, immersion, and absorption into an art process followed by emerging, reflecting, and narrating the process together with an observing witness. This "creative cycle" has been described in various ways by Ehrenzweig (1967), Schaverien (1992), Gordon (2000), Maclaggan (2001), McNiff (2004), and Franklin (2010). The creative cycle has two distinct phases that engage quite different internal processes: first, a sensory, physical, and body-oriented process experienced through the connection with arts media, movement, and expression and second, a process of reflection, observation, and cognition as both the therapist and the client conceptualise and articulate what has emerged through the creative act. I will consider both aspects of the creative cycle within an integrative arts therapy approach: first the art-making process and second the reflective, co-constructed articulation phase.

DOI: 10.4324/9781003155676-10

The sensory phase involves the movement of feelings and affects through visual arts media, using the sense of touch, movement, and sight, and is at the heart of an arts therapy experience. When we extend ourselves through creative and expressive acts and arts-based communication I find that we establish connectivity between the body, the psychological, and the imaginal experiences we have of ourselves. When this energetic movement is expressed through the visual arts, through making a mark, we begin to witness a tangible expression of affect, feeling, and meaning, a movement between the body and the mind, between the internal made visible. It is this externalising property of visual arts media that enables clients in art therapy to playfully examine a sense of identity in transition whilst opening to the potential of discovery through movement and creative expression.

Creative experiments

From the moment a client enters the art therapy studio, I notice the body, its gestural movements, and posture, as well as the energetic charge of the collaborative relationship. As I facilitate a movement from the presenting feeling and the client's narrative, I ask whether she might have an image or what the feeling being described might look like. This is always an invitation into art making and the beginning of a "creative experiment". Creative experiments begin as possibilities framed by curiosity and an open invitation to engage with the art materials. I might suggest larger or smaller paper or introduce a different medium or the use of clay. Sometimes I suggest standing up and fixing larger paper to the studio wall or to try working on the floor. These choices are all framed by safe, gradual experimentation based on phenomenological observation (Gilbert & Orlans, 2011) and collaborative choice-making and will be influenced by the responsiveness of the client in the present moment.

The term "experiment" is helpful when introducing a creative response in integrative arts psychotherapy, as a creative act is always full of potential, neither one of us knowing where it will take us. As a therapist, I sit back, attentively watching each mark, gesture, and movement as a visual form is given shape, direction, and rhythm, and the client's creative dance unfolds. The term "creative experiment" is used in gestalt therapy, and I find the definition given by Zinker (1978) inclusive of arts and acts to describe a movement from thinking to feeling through creativity.

Art externalises: a physical embodiment

In an art therapy session, the client is invited to reflect upon what is happening in their life and relationships, and the therapist listens. The client narrates their lived experience, and the therapist attunes to the rhythm and patterns that begin to form and dissolve and eventually crystalise into a poignant feeling or issue to work with in the session. This foreground concern or feeling is described as the "figure" as distinct from the "ground" of the client's phenomenological experience in gestalt theory (Joyce & Sills, 2008). Once the focus appears, the therapist typically facilitates several movements of energy. First, there is a movement into feeling and the emotional content aroused by the experience being described. This gives access to an emotional energy or the affect that the experience evokes through describing what is felt, where it is felt, and how it manifests itself in the physical body. The second movement is towards a creative act, also facilitated through the body as the therapist supports a choice of visual media that might give access to, and express, a particular feeling.

The physicality of art making generates a secondary sensation that may complement or amplify the feeling being expressed and worked with during the session. The experience of painting or mark-making involves touch, movement, friction, resistance, and flow; these are the "material qualities of painting" (Maclaggan, 2001). The physical contact between the hand and the material along with the kinetic energy required to make a mark and to develop it further requires movement that can mobilise a heightened experience of the feeling. Mark-making can be soothing, frustrating, flowing, or resisting. There may be a tension expressed by scraping, cutting, or by using abrasive or aggressive contact with the materials. The first vignette is an example of how the physicality of art making can support the expression of a feeling and generate a secondary sensation that may complement, amplify, and discharge an emotion.

Pru enters the session by describing feeling tension and frustration in relation to her husband, their shared life, and rising conflict between them. The feeling is located in the body, in her chest, in the same place as the hollow feelings of depression; it feels like there is anger "bottled-up" within the depressive feelings. I ask whether she might use the art materials to express the feeling, and she decides to use charcoal and conte on a large sheet of A1 paper (Figure 6.1). She chose to stand up and use the power of her body to press down on the paper. The materials generate hard jagged marks and a growing amount of pressure applied to the connective surface. The energy builds and intensifies until the image is felt to be complete. Both the client and the therapist pause, breathe, and look at the image together, we note the energy in the image and a change in energy towards the end of the process. It was this shift in energy that seemed significant and what happened visually on the page and what happened energetically in her body was explored further.

Pru reflected on the choice of materials, the mark-making, and the pace, tempo, and intensity experienced in making this image, she felt that it held and expressed the anger and aggression felt in her body. The shift in energy towards the end felt like a completion of the expression and opened a space to pause, to step back, and to breathe. This shift enabled another feeling to surface, along with a clarity and determination to change something in her relationship and to articulate the feeling rather than keeping it "bottled-up" in the body.

The creative art-making phase and experiment developed, intensified, and was experienced as completing itself when the energy peaked and then subsided. At this point, the client eased back from the image, and I guided the work into the

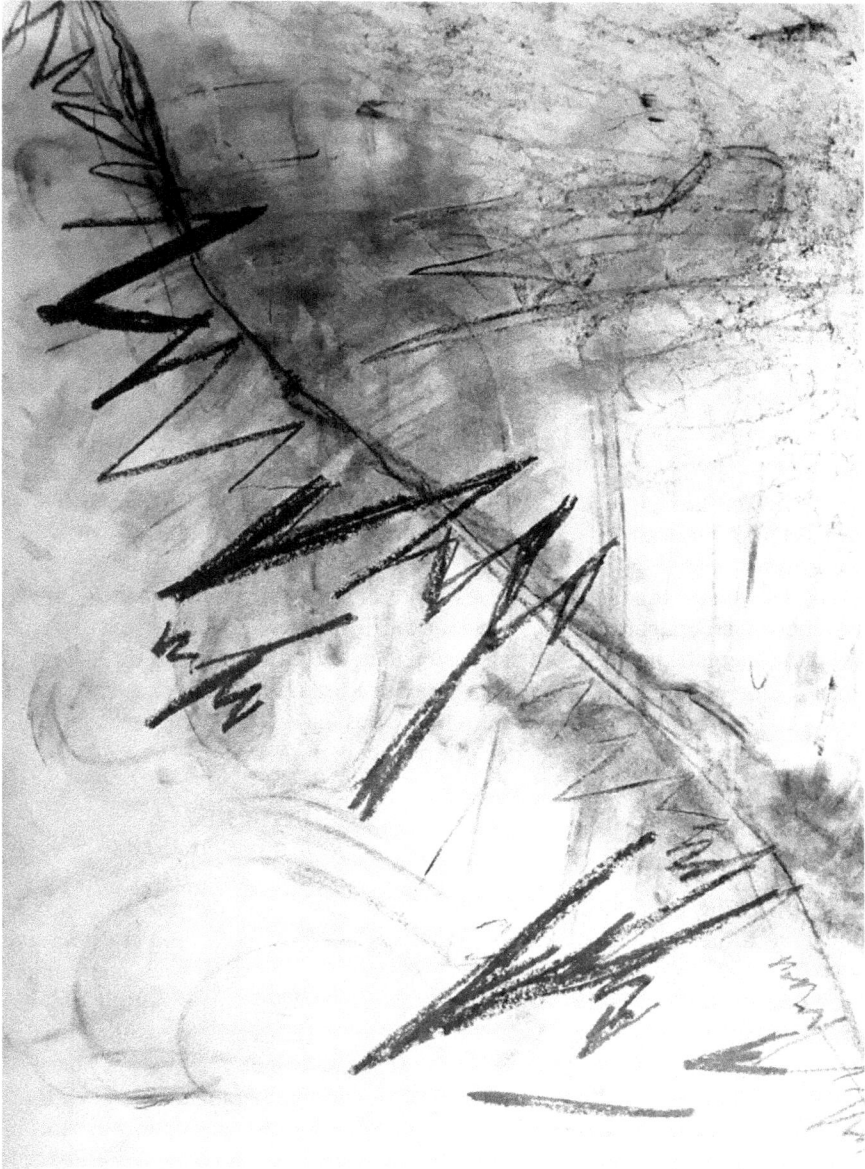

Figure 6.1 Crossing the line. Charcoal, pastel, and conte on paper

second phase of the creative cycle, a reflective narration of the experience. Both parts of the cycle occur within the receptive and respectful position facilitated through the "dialogic relationship" (Mann, 2010).

Creative healing: the dialogic relationship

Understanding the importance of the therapeutic relationship is central to the training and practice of art therapists as it is through the dynamic human encounter that the potential for change is mobilised. The practitioner's knowledge of human psychology and the movement of affect and imagination support this process, as does a "physiological theory of empathy" (Franklin, 2010), "art and intersubjectivity" (Skaife, 2001), "looking together and attunement" (Isserow, 2008), and "psychological aesthetics" (Maclaggan, 2001; McNiff, 2004). Within the relational work of therapy, it is the dialogue between an intersubjective experience of self and other that is held, imagined, and symbolically deepened through the expressive art form. This is achieved within the dialogic relationship described by Mackewn, (1997), Yontef and Levine Bar-Yoseph (2008), and Mann (2010), as a relational space in which therapists witness, accept unconditionally and absorb the client's expressive narratives and symbolic representations created through art. The dialogic relationship can be seen as an area within the therapeutic dyad where the creative language, objects, and images that are witnessed emerging achieve a quality of wonder and appreciation. It is the relational space in which the therapist and the client collaboratively mediate a change of viewpoint or perspective enabling the energetic quality of an expression to be fully accepted and valued. From this position creative presence is welcomed into the session, to be greeted as part of the client's psyche, to inform and influence psychological communication and give access to the potential for creative change to occur.

Shared viewing, witnessing, and completing the creative cycle

Whilst working with the visual narratives that emerge through the art object or image, as a therapist, I also witness the ways in which each unique expressive act leads to the creation of an image or artwork. As I observe each mark made, I am acutely aware of every hesitation or pause, and I gently absorb the waves of energy generated through each expressive gesture. Gradually, a composition develops, falls away, and then comes into focus. When an artwork has emerged and there is a sustained pause, both the client and the therapist draw back from the piece and move into a reflective, viewing position. As the focus moves from the act of art making into the feelings, mood, or expression contained in the artwork, I facilitate a collaborative exploration of what the client can see and how she experiences the image. The verbal narration of the visual content provides access to feeling and meaning through the abstract, lyrical associations evoked in response to the visual narrative language of art.

McNiff (2015) described the shared viewing of the artwork as completing the creative energetic cycle: "Successful artworks convey a sense of depth through presentational features evoking inner reverberations in the viewers and audiences who complete their expressive cycles and who are as necessary to creative vitality as artists are" (2015, p. 11). It is the shared viewing of the creative expression of another that contributes to the receptive and reflective phase within the creative cycle. Through a sustained looking at the art object, both the client and the therapist enter a period of attuned and active viewing that generates a focus of attention. This leads to collaboratively imagining further and deeper into the artwork, opening a playful and imaginative process of thinking together. Here new associations and creative links develop along with insights and possible meanings. This is a natural part of the cycle of immersion, creation, separation, reflection, and meaning-making that forms a core part of the therapy hour.

The process of active imagination can be used at this stage to access and deepen the therapeutic exploration of imagery. This may involve "dialoguing" with the image (McNiff, 1992), a process that engages verbally with the visual narrative through using the image, or part of the image, to ask what it might offer or communicate directly to the client or the therapist. Opening dialogue with the artwork allows symbolic resonances to emerge, and new metaphors or associations to take shape in the conversation between the client and their art supported and reflected by the therapist's facilitation approach. This is a further step in developing a creative experiment whereby we enter more fully into the dialogic engagement with creativity through the language of art and metaphor.

A movement into metaphor

The language of metaphor is essential to creative thinking, allowing us a capacity to play therapeutically with objects, images, and feelings. Metaphor allows one thing to stand for or reflect the qualities of something else, and for that thing being something difficult to put into words. In verbal psychotherapy, the use of metaphor opens up a playful space in which verbal language takes a detour away from the actual and into the realms of the possible. In the arts therapies, metaphor bridges the physical and aesthetic through a combination of visual, verbal, and kinaesthetic modes of communication, providing a conceptual link between the different language structures. In his work in "The role of metaphor in art therapy" (2007), Moon shows us that "[w]hen clients create an art piece, they gain access to the many layers of meaning contained in the metaphor at both conscious and unconscious levels" (p. 11).

The next case vignette describes how the movement between different language modes occurs as the image is extended into sculptural form and the use of space. Here metaphor is worked with to find connections between inner and outer experience, thus providing another bridge, this time between internal imagery and external articulation through the arts.

Spatial expression and three-dimensional construction of a developmental narrative

Suki is an arts therapy trainee and has been coming to therapy over the past two years. Personal therapy is part of the course requirement. Suki has been developing an interest in the use of shapes, construction, and the exploration of physical and relational space. She has just spent the weekend using sculptural materials as part of a workshop and brought the creative experience into the art therapy session. She constructs an assemblage of wire, string, plastic, and buttons and suspends them from a ceiling hook in the therapy room (Figure 6.2). She then takes paper, black paint, PVA, sticks, and wire and paints a thick, dark pond to represent something fearful and foreboding. Sitting between these two pieces, I listen to the client's narrative, speaking in part from the position of the artist describing her visual process; how it felt to make these pieces, and how one construction in the room led to the need to paint in another part of the room.

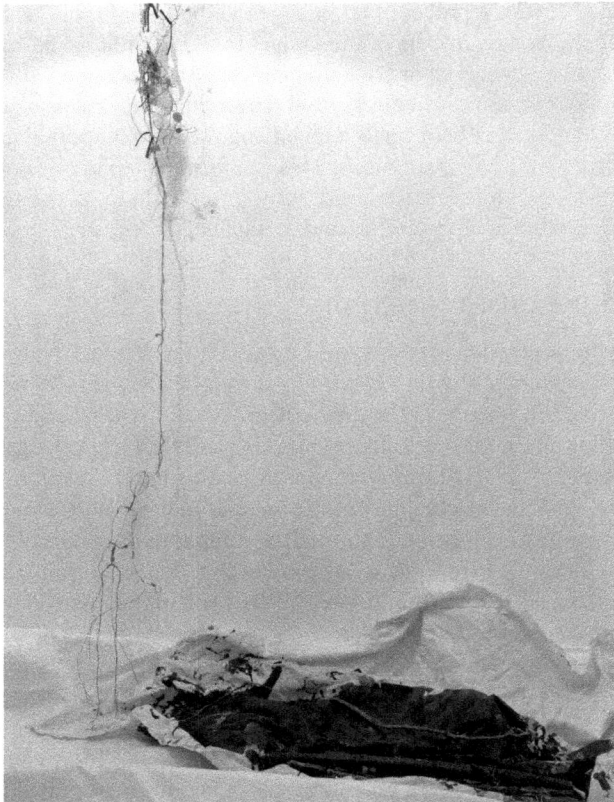

Figure 6.2 Wire, plastic, buttons, paper, glue, pigment, sticks, and earth

The movement between the two pieces is also described from the position of narrator of her internal process as she navigates her way from a safe, known, and reassuring use of familiar materials found in the construction and towards the fearful, frightening, and dark parts of self, memory, childhood, and the unconscious, as expressed through making the painting. The narration of the art-based experience takes the form of a story of "the secret garden", and the client becomes the storyteller of her own treacherous journey through therapy as she pieces together the fragments of her memories of childhood, adolescence, and the developmental milestones along the way.

A wire figure representing the client is placed between the two art pieces so as to show the size and scale of these places of "safety" and "fear". The feeling between us, between the artworks, the storyteller, and her therapist, resonates with the affective energy held within the story of the adult client entering the garden as a child. There is a sensitivity and tenderness as we slowly, cautiously, work with developmental trauma and fear.

The metaphoric language of art making, art objects, their creation, and assemblage in space are illustrated in this example. The internal narrative was given form through movement and projection onto objects and the construction of three-dimensional structures, followed by the imaginative development of the client's intrapsychic story of trauma and loss. Within the framed space of arts psychotherapy, and within the language of metaphor, a creative act was facilitated using the vocabulary of the chosen arts media to articulate what it is to be and to communicate this felt experience to a witnessing therapist.

Facilitating attention towards creative expression

As we work with and through the artwork, I look for creative ways to support clients to elaborate or amplify the many references, associations, and possible meanings flowing through an image. Metaphor provides an access point, a hook into thinking, allowing a space in which to freely associate with the artwork and to play with meaning as we explore what a colour, shape, texture, or composition might stand for or point towards. In arts psychotherapy sessions, I frequently ask the simple question: what would a feeling, thought, memory, or experience look like? Or could you make an image in response to that particular tension in your body or conflict you are describing? Once made, the visual image or clay piece often suggests other verbal associations. When we sit back and view the piece thoughtfully, playfully, together, something new, often unexpected, emerges. Words form to capture what is seen and quite often a metaphor arises that seems to hold more than the client or the therapist was initially aware of. The visual form is then available to both the client and the therapist to view, reflect, and honour. I may then suggest that we explore and develop further associations in relation to the content of the image on the page by extending the metaphors in the imagery into expressive body movement and gesture.

In the creative arts therapies (music, drama, dance, movement, and the visual arts), the use of metaphor is elaborated and amplified through each different creative medium using movement, rhythm, melody, enactment, image, or sculpted form. Informed by drama and body-oriented therapies, an integrative approach places an emphasis on the body and a greater focus upon how the body itself may hold, move, and express metaphor. Dramatherapy methods encourage participants to "embody the metaphor" by feeling the metaphor and expressing it through the "dramatic body" (Jones, 2007). This is achieved by dramatic stance, posture, gesture, and the enactment of the emerging metaphoric narrative as it is felt and expressed through the physical and energetic body of the client.

I have found that "embodying" the metaphor can be used to transition between a feeling in the body and the image on the page. As the client's creative flow progresses, I may extend the creative experiment by focusing on body awareness and drawing attention to the breath and the "felt sense" as described by Rappaport (2009). This gentle shift in awareness locates a feeling in the body and moves it into art making. The method encourages a connection between what the body feels and how the body might use creative media to express a particular feeling.

From the body into metaphor into the arts

Two parallel processes emerge when using the arts to work with metaphoric imagery that originates in bodily feeling. First, the feeling in the body is explored in terms of sensation, movement, and gesture, and second, it is explored visually as a textural image in the mind of the client and/or the therapist. These two processes demonstrate a link between internal bodily sensations and how the senses then contribute to imagining the feeling and externalising the experience through an art form.

The first process refers to body sensation or "vitality affects" (Stern, 1998) that may be felt and described as a churning, vibrating, pulsing, swaying, trembling, wrenching, burning, tingling, numbing, aching, or throbbing feeling. The sensation can then be developed by describing a movement such as stillness, frozen, static, inert, blocked, melting, flowing, fluttering, a moving towards or away from, running, leaping, flying, or falling. The second process draws on the sense of sight and visualisation by developing an internal image that holds or reflects something of the feeling experienced in the body. Using visual adjectives to extend the "look" of the feeling and to describe whether it is light or dark, rough, jagged, pointed, sharp or smooth, soft, comforting, or smothering, we transpose body sensation into visual metaphor.

The movement from bodily sensation into visual metaphor is followed by using the senses to communicate what the body is feeling in the moment. I support the client to bring "presence" to the therapeutic process by attending to the "felt sense" experienced in the here and now. In verbal psychotherapy, the formation of imaginative verbal associations provides a playful, creative space in which imagery, pattern, form, and feeling are explored through metaphor. When the arts are introduced, the therapist facilitates the emergence of metaphor through the communication mode that the client is feeling and sensing at the moment. In integrative arts psychotherapy, the invitation is to use arts media to externalise the image located in the body. The physiological feeling may be expressed with body movement, using the visual sense to form an image, or the sound of the sensation may be amplified and repeated to experience the resonance of sound improvisation in the room and in the body.

When combining metaphors drawn from the body with a movement into art making, I find that the dramatic expression informs the visual imagery as body movement is transposed into the creative art form. When this occurs, there is potential to support the client to step into and embody the metaphor on the page, to explore the feeling content through visual media and the verbal associations that arise. The reverse process is also possible by encouraging the client to lift the metaphor off the page and allow it to find expression through the body in the form of gestural expression, vocal sound, or body rhythm, thus experiencing the metaphoric language of art through the body. The different art forms can then be harnessed to find the expressive language that best communicates the feeling, affect, or narrative held by the metaphor. This might be through movement, sound, rhythm, voice, action, or sculpting. They are then woven into verbal narratives or extended into story or poetic prose and rhythm.

Endings and reviews: the retrospective review

Images and artworks hold many different meanings, and their metaphoric value can change over time as our perceptions of them alter and our perspective of the context in which they were made also changes. The visual arts, sandtray, and performance arts increasingly use digital recordings of the enactments, sculptural artworks, and sandtray scenarios. The tangible art object or digital photographic record captures a trace of the therapeutic journey, and in art therapy, the review of the images is known as a "retrospective review" (Schaverien, 1993). This is a point in art therapy when the client and the therapist mutually instigate a review of the artwork: "The retrospective review of a series of pictures which demonstrates progress and changes which have taken place over days, weeks, months and even years" (1993, p. 33). Schaverien suggests that it is during the review of the artwork that clients have a unique opportunity to "see" their therapeutic journey revealed through their art. The review, whether it occurs at intervals in therapy or during the ending process, always produces new connections, narration, and meaning as artworks connect and widen their metaphoric reference points from one image to the next.

Manoj arranges his paintings across the studio floor, this is artwork from one full year of art therapy and so they fill the room (Figure 6.3). The images are laid out chronologically, and as we stand back to look at the full visual impact of the work, certain images come into focus and others recede. Both the client and the therapist notice an early image of a figure in the mist resonate with a later

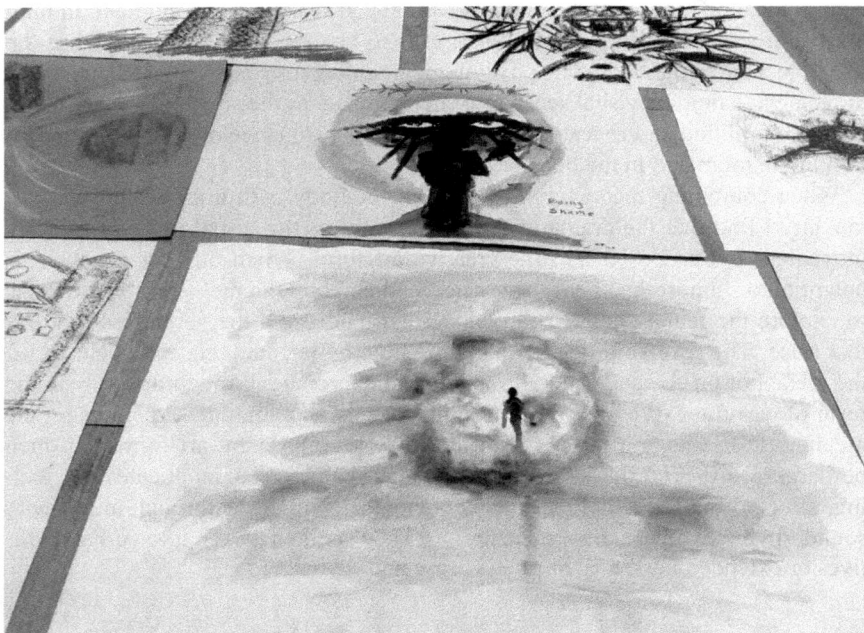

Figure 6.3 Retrospective review

image of a figure walking towards the viewer as though it could be the same figure of a young man emerging from the mist. These two images then resonate with a third, a more recent image of a full portrait of a face looking out of the picture.

Each image had its own particular visual and verbal narrative and associations from the time and context in which it was made, one narrative was the exploration of self, identity, cultural difference, social isolation, and facing oneself in therapy. When viewed together, the three images gave a visual representation of a central therapeutic narrative, that of personal discovery, change, and transition during the journey of therapy and training to become a therapist. What became apparent in the third image was that the visual narrative shows the client confronting an aspect of self that was reflected back through the portrait image, as if a visual mirror was held up to reflect a part of the client's identity that is formed from and discovered within his creativity.

The retrospective review has become an integral process in art therapy and is used across all client groups and contexts. It is also an opportunity for the client to reflect on his or her experience of the therapy and the relational process that can bring a potential for levelling the power relationship. In practice, the combination of what is seen and sensed in the other is extended and amplified, verified, or dismissed during a retrospective review. It can then be used to modify or focus the course of ongoing therapeutic work (Springham, 2016; Nash, 2018) and acts as a tangible metaphoric container for the therapeutic journey for each client at the end of the therapy relationship.

Conclusion

Integrative arts psychotherapy brings together a range of arts media and the potential to move through a creative cycle in the fullness of the timeframe of an individual or groupwork session. In this chapter, I have shown how I encourage clients who are able to trust in the therapeutic relationship and feel safe enough with me to articulate their experience so that we can work collaboratively and co-design creative and therapeutic processes.

My facilitation approach is informed by what the client presents in the moment as I seek to guide the experience towards an exploration of what is implied, an expression of what might be imagined, or a creative response towards what a particular narrated experience might look, sound, or feel like. The choice of media can deepen or amplify the material being expressed, and the different art forms used can mediate a movement of unspoken, physiological, and psychological energy. The physicality involved when making art enables clients to feel present and access the kinetic energy of the body through mark-making, mixing media, or manipulating clay. There is also an aesthetic energy that is activated through colour relationship, the movement of paint or dry materials, and the emergence of form. The visual form resonates with the free-associative capacity of visual perception, and when the controls are relaxed enough, a creative flow or playful energy can be released.

The expressive art form, image, or object that emerges provides containment of this expression. When an image has been made, there is an opportunity to dialogue with it, and in so doing, we step into the metaphoric language provided by the artwork by supporting the client to amplify and articulate their relationship with the image, embody the metaphor, and complete the creative cycle.

References

Clarkson, P. (1989) *The therapeutic relationship*. London: Whurr Publishers.

Ehrenzweig, A. (1967) *The hidden order of art: A study in the psychology of artistic imagination*. London: Weidenfeld & Nicolson.

Franklin, M. (2010) Affect regulation, mirror neurons, and the third hand: Formulating mindful empathic art interventions. *Art Therapy: Journal of the American Art Therapy Association, 27 (4), pp. 160–167.*

Gilbert, M. & Orlans, V. (2011) *Integrative therapy: 100 key points and techniques*. Hove and New York: Routledge.

Gordon, R. (2000) *Dying and creating: A search for meaning*. London: Karnac Books Ltd.

Isserow, I. (2008) Looking together: Joint attention in art therapy. *International Journal of Art Therapy, 13 (1), pp. 34–42.*

Jones, P. (2007) *Drama as therapy: Theory, practice and research* (second edition). Hove and New York: Routledge.

Joyce, P. & Sills, C. (2008) *Skills in gestalt counselling and psychotherapy*. Los Angeles, London, New Delhi and Singapore: Sage.

Mackewn, J. (1997) *Developing gestalt counselling*. London: Sage.

Maclaggan, D. (2001) *Psychological aesthetics: Painting, feeling and making sense*. London and Philadelphia: Jessica Kingsley Publications.

Mann, D. (2010) *Gestalt therapy: 100 key points and techniques*. Hove and New York: Routledge.

McNiff, S. (1992) *Art as medicine: Creating a therapy of the imagination*. Boston, London: Shambhala Publications.

McNiff, S. (2004) *Art heals: How creativity cures the soul*. Boston: Shambhala Publications.

McNiff, S. (2015) *Imagination in action: Secrets for unleashing creative expression*. Boston: Shambhala Publications.

Moon, B. (2007) *The role of metaphor in art therapy: Theory, method and experience*. Springfield, IL: Charles C. Thomas Publisher.

Nash, G. (2018) Evaluation and review of art psychotherapy in private practice. *International Journal of Art Therapy, 23 (1), pp. 25–32.* http://dx.doi.org/10.1080/17454832.2017.1323934

Rappaport, L. (2009) *Focusing-oriented art therapy: Accessing the body's wisdom and creative intelligence*. London and Philadelphia: Jessica Kingsley Publishers.

Schaverien, J. (1992) *The revealing image: Analytical art psychotherapy in theory and practice*. London and Philadelphia: Jessica Kingsley Publishers.

Schaverien, J. (1993) The retrospective review of pictures: Data for research in art therapy. In H. Payne (ed.), *Handbook of inquiry in the arts therapies: One river, many currents*, pp. 91–103. London and Bristol: Jessica Kingsley Publications.

Springham, N. (2016) Description as social construction in UK art therapy research. *International Journal of Art Therapy, 21 (3), pp. 104–115.*

Skaife, S. (2001) Making visible: Art therapy and intersubjectivity. *International Journal of Art Therapy, 6 (2), pp. 40–50.*

Stern, D. (1998) *The interpersonal world of the infant: A view from psychoanalysis and developmental psychology*. London: Karnac Books.

Yontef, G. & Levine Bar-Yoseph, T. (2008) Dialogic relationship – Chapter 9. In Brownell, P. (ed.), *Handbook for theory, research and practice in gestalt therapy*, pp. 184–197. Newcastle: Cambridge Scholars Publishing.

Zinker, J. (1978) *Creative process in gestalt therapy*. New York; Toronto: Vintage Books.

Chapter 7

Embodied sound

Voicing the voiceless self

Hannah Rees

Introduction

In this chapter, I explore the role of the *sung voice* in arts psychotherapy, as an embodied practice with a trauma-informed approach. Vocalisation and the sung voice are untapped resources in arts psychotherapy, remaining largely unexplored as vehicles for improvisation. The creative therapeutic potential of music is one of the seven art forms used at the Institute of Arts in Therapy and Education.

Within the field of music therapy, Diane Austin has pioneered working with the voice through "songs of self", and her model of vocal psychotherapy is now well known (Austin, 2008). I consider three ways in which voicework can be used in arts psychotherapy, using case examples. I demonstrate how the latest findings in trauma research can underpin voicework with clients impacted by complex trauma; how the sung voice, as the most intimate expression of our relationship to self, can be an immediate way of accessing wounded, even pre-verbal parts of the client that have remained silent for a long time; and how, by bringing them into vocal expression, those parts previously alienated from the self can be welcomed and befriended – creating a new, self-sounding narrative.

I use the formulation *sung voice* (Goodchild, 2015) to differentiate the concept from that of the traditional "singing" voice, which carries a heavy burden of expectations and conditioning. It tends to be viewed as the preserve of those with formal training rather than as our common birthright, celebrating what makes us human. Approaching the voice in this way also helps connect us to the vocalising creativity of infants and children, who naturally sing to themselves as they acquire language.

I propose that trauma-informed voicework in arts psychotherapy is the therapeutic use of voice, namely, breathing, natural sounds, toning, vocalisation, and improvisational singing within the client–therapist dyad. At the heart of this work is the healing relationship, with insights from the Six Therapeutic Relationships Framework (Gilbert & Orlans, 2010) used to reflect on and plan for the therapeutic journey uniquely with each client. This also supports the therapist to consider risk and to grade and pace interventions with care, taking account of these different relationships. I work collaboratively with my clients, enquiring into their

DOI: 10.4324/9781003155676-11

relationship to music and singing so as to enable them to bring into our work their own cultural background and traditions of using voice and song.

The therapist develops a good working alliance with the client and creates a safe environment that can vocally contain the client's expressive sound. She also teaches practices that allow the client to stabilise in the present, including using their voice to recruit the "social engagement system". Dyadic improvised singing can facilitate a process whereby unexplored feeling states or disowned wounded parts from trauma can be accessed and expressed. Dyadic improvisational singing involves the therapist lending her own voice, sometimes accompanied by a drum, Shruti box, ukulele, or harmony instrument, and inviting the client to put their feelings into sound through vocalising and improvised singing together. Within the attuned therapeutic dyad, the client can allow those younger, previously disowned parts to be heard, owned, and brought home to the self.

"Safe and Sound": Polyvagal Theory, breathing, toning, and the safe place

According to safe trauma treatment (Herman, 1992; Rothschild, 2000; Fisher, 1999), it is paramount to create an environment of safety for the client, one where they feel safe to make sounds. In order to grasp this more fully, we need to consider some of the latest findings in neurobiology and Polyvagal Theory, in particular the research of Dr Stephen Porges, which offers an advanced understanding of the autonomic nervous system (ANS), especially as regards trauma and PTSD (Porges, 2011).

The ANS is regulated by the vagus nerve or tenth cranial nerve, which connects the brain to major systems in the body, supporting mind–body communications. Mammals have two vagal circuits, an evolutionarily older "dorsal vagal complex" and a more recently evolved "ventral vagal complex", also referred to as the "social engagement system". The dorsal vagal complex connects to the organs underneath the diaphragm including the stomach, spleen, liver, kidneys, as well as the small and large intestines. The ventral vagal, social engagement system connects above the diaphragm to the heart, lungs, larynx, pharynx, inner ear, as well as the facial muscles around the mouth and eyes.

Generally speaking, the vagus nerve is associated with the parasympathetic nervous system and has an inhibitory influence upon the heart and sympathetic nervous system activity. Most importantly, Porges's (2011) research has identified that the parasympathetic nervous system has two presentations depending upon whether one feels safe or threatened. In times of safety, the parasympathetic nervous system facilitates rest, relaxation, and digestion. However, in times of threat, the parasympathetic nervous system has a defensive mode. How might vocalisation and sounding contribute to regulating the mind–body communications mediated by the vagus nerve?

The foundation of support in stimulating the vagus nerve and activating physiological state shifts is *self-regulation* through grounding the body, anchoring the breath, and vocalisation. Before the client is ready to engage in using their voice and sharing it with the therapist in the psychotherapeutic space, the therapist's own voice is vital for signalling safety. As Deb Dana (2018: 146) suggests, "a voice with appropriate patterns of rhythm and sound invites the listener into safe connection". Prosody, the variations in vocal stress and intonation communicate what lies beneath the words, conveying the speaker's emotional state and intention (Belyk & Brown, 2016).

However, using the voice to express feelings in the moment is particularly exposing, as it reminds us how inextricably linked our sense of self is to the sound of our voice. Judgements, criticisms, and apologies can flood the client, touching on the wounded self that was deemed "not good enough" or unacceptable in the eyes of others. Acknowledging the "inner critic" within clients who have experienced trauma or traumatic attachment, the act of making a sound and giving themselves a voice can evoke how often they have felt compelled to silence that voice in order to stay safe. My aim is to foster an environment that acknowledges the "nakedness" (Goodchild, 2015) the client may feel when making such a sound, notwithstanding any previous singing experience.

It takes courage to sing!

The courage to find and use the sung voice can be developed by grounding the client in their body; a sense of safety and security begins with an awareness of where the feet are on the ground, enabling orientation. Working up from here using exercises borrowed from yoga, Alexander Technique, Feldenkreis, and other traditions of movement helps the client sink into their body-self by connecting to their body's strength along with vocalisations such as yawning and sighing. Additional natural sounds produced spontaneously by our voices, such as laughing, moaning, wailing, and grunting, are explored along with the involuntary movements of the body corresponding to them.

By way of example, let us consider Alexander's monkey position, which is voiced. Here the legs bend slightly at the knees, the pelvis tilts forwards, the space under the arms increases, the physiognomy relaxes, the eyes lose specific focus, the jaw drops passively, the tongue falls forwards onto the bottom lip, the pharyngeal space falls open, and the larynx descends in the neck to allow a sense of the throat opening (Newham, 1998: 162–163). In this position, the client is encouraged to make the "neutral schwa" sound as in "ago" (phonetic symbol "ə"). This engages the body and connects it to the voice. This exercise is key to building up trust in making an embodied sound.

Breathing, the foundation for an embodied sound, provides further stabilisation, laying the basis for the next stage. The exercise I find most helpful – I call it "Three breaths out" – involves extending the outbreath as long as possible, so that, with practice, the back muscles become activated. This practice can be enhanced by asking the client to include a second's pause before drawing breath again. This exercise can be very effective in stimulating the vagus nerve and creating a state shift from the sympathetic to the ventral vagal state. It "results in short inhalations and extended durations of exhalations . . . breathing increases the calming impact and health benefits of the myelinated vagus on our body" (Porges, 2011: 253–254). As such, breath practice anticipates the energising and calming impact that singing can have on the nervous system and reduces inhibitions around vocalisation by recruiting the ventral vagal system in a more supportive body connection. The client will now feel more grounded in their body to support their voice in making embodied sounds such as toning, vocalisation, and improvisational singing.

Toning

Toning is the creation of a sustained, often non-verbal vocal sound, the audible vibration of breath heard in vowel sounds aah, ayy, eeh, ohh, ooh. If toning feels too challenging, this exercise can be calibrated by starting with humming or blowing through a Kazoo. As an active body intervention, toning or humming is a useful meditation alternative because, by being invited to make an audible vibration, the client attends to the sound rather than their thoughts. This can be particularly effective in increasing vagal tone, especially when eye contact may be too challenging for clients holding a lot of trauma. According to Peper et al.'s research study (2019), toning is a "useful strategy to reduce mind wandering and intrusive thoughts" (p. 132), as well as to slow the respiration rate and increase heart-rate variability, two factors in measuring emotional and physiological self-regulation and achieving sympathetic and parasympathetic balance.

A variation on the toning exercise is for the client and the therapist to sound together, either with the eyes closed or at least without making eye contact. The traumatised client may find eye contact particularly triggering, as trauma can turn off the social engagement system (Porges, 2011: 252). For clients who might otherwise find themselves poised for fight or flight in the therapeutic setting (i.e., experiencing a high heart rate and low vagal regulation of the heart), toning together can therefore be a very stabilising intervention, helping to increase vagal tone.

Safe place, self-boundary, and voicework

Creating a safe space as a way of establishing inner safety is key for the client grappling with confusing, conflicting emotions and sensations that feel "too much" or "too little". A useful exercise to help stabilise the client is the "Tangible Boundary Exercise" from Sensorimotor Psychotherapy (Ogden & Fisher 2015: 411) in combination with voicework, allowing the client to experiment with putting a physical boundary around themselves. The therapist invites the client to tone in the space and fill it with their vibrations, so creating an additional sonic boundary.

Imagining an oasis of calm in their private sanctuary, the client can experience feeling safe with themselves and their inner experience. I have developed the Safe Place exercise by combining it with the sung voice. The therapist invites the client to tune into the sound of their inner calm and resonating silence and to listen out for the sound associated with their sanctuary, by sounding and toning, improvising a melody, or recalling a song known to them. The client is asked what they might need from the therapist to vocalise the sound that is resonating and is offered a menu of options. Sometimes vocalising can feel like creating more layers of protection or even a barrier of sound between the client and the outside. If it is a familiar song, we explore the client's relationship to that song.

Case example – "Golden Light"

Jenny, a 50-year-old white female, presented in my private practice with low mood, anxiety, and low self-esteem. She felt worthless in the eyes of her mother. She was haunted by a feeling that life was passing her by. My clinical thinking included developmental trauma as she struggled to hold herself in mind.

In Jenny's case, we had done the safe place exercise a while before and the beautiful scene of being drenched in warm, golden light offering endless possibilities of living a full life returned as a motif in therapy a number of times. In a previous session, she had drawn the scene (Figure 7.1), which then became the basis for an improvised song without words which she called "Golden Light".

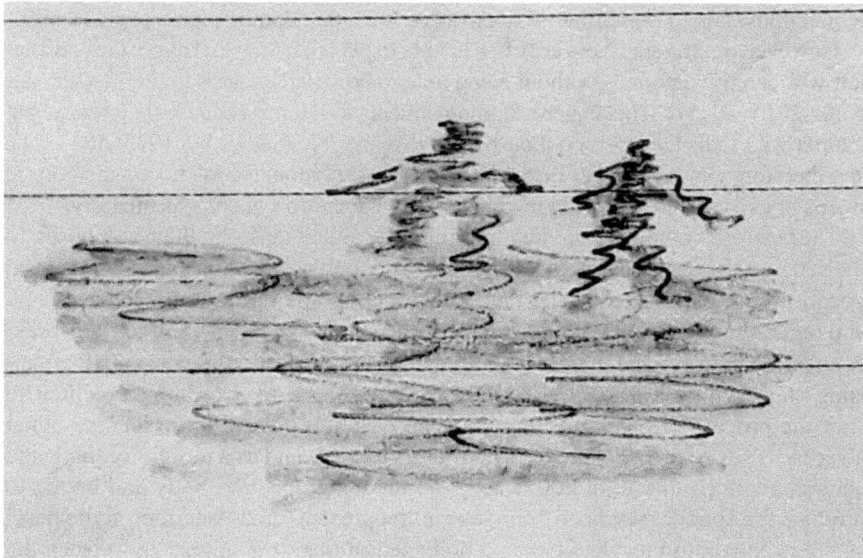

Figure 7.1 Golden light. Pencil, pen, and crayon on paper

The improvisation began with Jenny's gentle movement in response to the waves of light in the picture and then swaying back and forth in her seat to mirror the fluidity of the figure. I carefully mirrored her movements and we started to entrain together. I offered some sounds and invited her to join in, echoing some of her musical phrases. As soon as Jenny's voice gained confidence in rhythm and melody, I dropped in volume and pitch and sang a drone-like accompaniment to her ever-expanding phrases.

Using movement, breath, image, and sound can be a powerful and memorable intervention, which ultimately embeds the safe place exercise more deeply. After mobilising the body and firing up the imagination, making a sound and vocalising in this intermodal approach can be particularly containing for a client who feels not only inhibited about using their voice but also fearful of vocal improvisation in the therapy session.

Meeting aspects of self through song

In this section, I propose that therapeutic voicework in arts psychotherapy can enable the client to tap into feeling states of their traumatic past through "improvised dyadic singing without words", a form of non-verbal vocalising between the client and the therapist. The practice of improvised dyadic singing without words allows feeling states to be accessed which may otherwise remain silent. Schore's extensive work (2003) has established that these feeling states are held in the right-brain hemisphere in implicit memory, which is unconscious, non-verbal, and relational. Implicit memory is not subject to direct recall, unlike explicit memory, which allows us to remember in a narrative form that can be expressed verbally.

However, trauma survivors are often unable to put what they feel into words and are left with intense emotions without being able to articulate what is going on (Van der Kolk, 2014: 50–51). This is hard for many clients to fathom because they remember trauma with their feelings and their bodies (Van der Kolk & Fisler, 1995: 505–521), and therefore experience it as occurring in the present moment. Without a memory in words or even pictures, they do not recognise what they are feeling as memory.

Therapeutic voicework invites the client to make sense of their responses to their traumatic past, by putting feelings and body sensations into non-verbal vocalisations, supported by the therapist vocally, moment by moment, in a safe and regulating way. Safety and regulation are ensured by right-brain to right-brain connection between the therapist and the client. As a result, the non-verbal vocalising stays within a small range. Therapeutic voicework can help the client to start the process of distinguishing between past and present by practicing "dual awareness" as a "prerequisite for safe trauma therapy and as a tool for braking and containment" (Rothschild, 2000: 129). As the client engages body and breath to produce the sound, they keep "one foot in the present" and "one foot in the past" as they connect to their feelings and body sensations. It is important to teach the client that "feelings and sensations are the best guides for interpreting past reality", and that mindful awareness is a way of staying in the present.

Making space for silence and inviting the client to check in with their body-self, especially before vocalisation, are key. As Malchiodi (2020: 62) argues, "Silence is a factor in how expressive arts enhance the ability to 'look inside' oneself through interoception (the sense of the body's internal state) and experience a 'felt sense' of what is perceived and sensed in one's body".

"Felt Sense"

The concept of the "felt sense" is central to focusing, a mind/body practice developed by Gendlin (1996) which accesses an integrated, embodied knowing in the present moment. As Rappaport says, "listening to the felt sense opens the doorway to the body's wisdom – bringing next steps towards growth and healing" (2009: 23). For the traumatised client, focusing on their felt sense is akin to hearing their "instinctual voice", which provides a "backdrop for reconnecting with the animal in ourselves", as Peter Levine, the proponent of Somatic Experiencing, describes in "Waking the Tiger" (1997: 86).

Creating the space to allow the client to vocalise the instinctual sounds of their human animal self by accessing their felt sense can be a profound and healing experience, as in Lana's case later.

Vocalising the felt sense – case example

The work with private practice client Lana, a 33-year old, white European, centred on her longing to be in a relationship despite her fear of men and intimacy following the traumatic, violent assault by her ex-boyfriend in her 20s.

Lana arrived saying that she felt triggered by going on dates and that her throat felt "strangled and weak". She said that she wanted to do some voicework to ground herself. I gradually put the following felt sense questions to her: just notice the sensations in your throat, welcome and be friendly to them. Are some sensations subtle, and some stronger? Is there a rhythm to the sensations?

She said that she felt sad. I asked her if there was a sound that matched her felt sense of sadness and she made some whimpering noises with her lips tightly pressed together.

I asked if I could join in, and as she glanced at the Shruti box, I offered to play some chords similar in pitch to the sounds she was making. Mirroring the sustained chords, we started humming together and she made eye contact.

Aware of my countertransference of wanting to cry, I invited the client to vocalise open vowel sounds by releasing her jaw slightly. I offered less volume but toned with her as her voice gained in strength, toning long "uuuh" sounds. These then became higher pitched "aaahuuhh" sounds. As her diaphragm moved more rapidly, she released into tearful crying which then ebbed away.

In this case, vocalising the felt sense supported the release of deep sadness and the body's wisdom to express this naturally by involuntary crying and the realisation that she "strangled" her sadness. "The goal is to help the person not only release this 'stuck energy', but also redirect that energy into an active response" (Malchiodi, 2020: 206).

Words let me down – case example

Jenny longed to be free to be herself in relationships with others but felt held back by a fear of rejection and disapproval. She kept herself small and under the radar, having given up on having a voice in the world. Her relationship with her unresponsive and dismissive mother left her feeling deeply ashamed of her "unlived" life.

Voicework helped her access these feeling states of shame and self-loathing. She found non-verbal improvised singing profoundly freeing and intensely moving. This involved a co-regulating musical duet that replicates the "dyadic dance" (Schore, 2001) or, as I prefer, improvised "dyadic song" between the mother and the infant mentioned earlier. As a result, she was able to stay with her feelings and voice in song her fear, shame, and sadness, which she had been working so hard to hide, rather than rejecting or minimising these feelings.

> Steele, Boon and Van der Hart (2017: 310) refer to "hidden shame" and that this "hiding may be conscious, but much more often shame is simply outside the awareness of patients, who have managed to hide it so thoroughly from themselves that they cannot recall the memories that sustain in."

I realised that this allowed Jenny to take her feelings seriously, to treat herself differently from how her mother had done, and to validate her own experience. Through her tears, she resolutely exclaimed: "Words let me down!" For Jenny, words meant confusion and conflict in making herself understood. She had learnt that it was better "not to say" what she wanted or needed in order to keep the peace. Through the process of therapeutic song making, she was able to challenge her perception of herself as somebody worthless who therefore "had nothing to say".

Once the client has found their way through the barrier of inhibition around making vocalised sounds in front of the therapist, improvised dyadic singing can be a non-threatening way of emerging from hiding and daring to express what was previously disowned, censored, diminished, or too painful to put into words. This vocalising activity provides a vehicle of expression beyond words, bypassing symbolic language, enabling the client to "feel" aspects of their traumatised past and experience the relief of translating these feelings into musical sound.

Expansion of the self and befriending the child self

In this section, I explore how voicework can help clients who have experienced trauma or wounds of attachment to access disowned aspects of themselves that have been split off due to trauma-related fragmentation and dissociation and to allow young, wounded internal states to be heard and befriended through vocalisation and improvised dyadic singing.

In trauma-related fragmentation, dissociation is the brain's and body's survival strategy for dealing with an overwhelming threat. According to the model known as Structural Dissociation, developed by Van der Hart, Nijenhuis and Steele (2006), the right-brain side of the self – named the "Traumatized Part of the Personality" – holds the feelings and body memories and the fearful expectation that the trauma will happen again. It stands on guard, poised for danger, and focused on threat. In this model, the left-brain side of the self is called the "Apparently Normal Part of the Personality", and it carries on with normal life, often with little or no memory of what happened. This part is focused on what needs to be done today.

Janina Fisher (2017: 19–32) emphasises the importance of helping clients to think about distress as communication from a traumatised child part and to engage in "speaking the language of parts" (2017: 8). This heightens their awareness that the overwhelming feeling from the past is a part of the self, wishing to make itself heard and not the whole self. Rather than over-identifying with the traumatised part to the detriment of the apparently normal part, we meet it with interest and curiosity, so activating the attentive brain and remaining mindfully in the present.

The struggle song – case example

Jenny was feeling an intense sense of shame and worthlessness and told me about her "inability to get a foothold in the adult world without fear of tripping up", i.e., her difficulty finding a new career in which she would take satisfaction and feel valued. When asked how old this fearful and ashamed part of her was, she replied: "six" and described herself as in touch with a general feeling of being ignored and not mattering. Asked what she wanted to say to her child part that was making herself known, she said that she could see she was struggling. I invited her to sing about her struggle and offered a menu of options to help locate herself in pitch and tone, such as the Shruti box, mini piano, and drum. She opted for minor chords and after I started to tone to these, Jenny joined me and soon branched off into a number of riffs which she repeated and embellished. Then she latched onto the word "struggle" and a song of struggle began to take shape.

The Struggle Song

Oh, it is always a struggle to be me *(client's voice)*
Such a struggle to be me *(therapist's voice)*
Oh, oh, it is always such a struggle to be me *(client's voice)*
Such a struggle to be me *(therapist's voice)*
Always such a struggle to be me *(client's voice) (repeated several times)*
Such a struggle to be free. *(client's voice)*

As I tuned into my counter-transference, I felt a longing to be set free rising in my chest and an impulse to raise my arms as if to unshackle myself. Jenny's song of struggle seemed to represent her sense of oppression, enslaved by the enmeshment with her primary caregivers, and of deep sadness. Improvised dyadic singing allowed that young, wounded part of herself to come out and be heard. As she heard herself sing of her struggle, the client told me of her grief at being unable to admit to these feelings previously. Struck by Jenny's ability now to own her feelings, after witnessing her own voice amplified by dyadic singing, I wondered about her song of struggle as an act of resistance.

Singing from the traumatised child part can often be the first time that the client allows themselves to get in touch with and express this "voiceless" part of themselves. The invitation to sing enables them to make contact with their feelings, "feel" aspects of their traumatised past, and own them as integral parts of their being. As the child part allows their singing to be followed by a silent, deep listening, the client begins to hear themselves, to be heard, and to feel safe (Fisher, 2017). This feeling of safety enables them to widen their "window of tolerance" (Siegel, 1999) and to be less overwhelmed by aspects of their traumatic past or by communication with others. By choosing to incorporate words into their improvised singing, the client signals a developmental stage where they can now access the reflective and communicative capacities of their adult self.

Conclusion – coming home

I have illustrated how trauma-informed voicework in integrative arts psychotherapy can enable wounded, traumatised parts of the client to come home and be fostered back into the family of self. The possibility of healing occurs as these parts are soothed by regulating vocalisation and improvised dyadic singing, which transforms their pain into punchy protest songs or beautifully touching lullabies. The connection with the self can be restored as new bonds are nurtured. The trauma survivor, no longer alienated from themselves, can create a new self-sounding narrative of self-acceptance and sing their "new reality" (Storr, 1997) into existence, often feeling uplifted and joyful as they harness their life force through the activity of singing.

As Herman (1992) tells us: "*Trauma dehumanizes the victim, the group restores her humanity . . . mirrored in the actions of others, the survivor recognizes and reclaims a lost part of herself. At that moment, the survivor begins to re-join the human commonality*" (p. 118).

As the trauma survivor reclaims their sung voice in therapy, they can feel more empowered to make themselves heard among their peers, intimate others, family members, work colleagues, and the wider community. Autonomy and agency mark their healing journey of joyfully coming home to their embodied sound and voicing their voiceless self.

References

Austin, D. (2008). *The theory and practice of vocal psychotherapy: Songs of the self.* London and Philadelphia: Jessica Kingsley Publishers.

Belyk, M., & Brown, S. (2016). Pitch underlies activation of the vocal system during affective vocalization. *Social Cognitive and Affective Neuroscience,* 11 (7), 1078–1088. DOI: 10.1093/scan/nsv074

Dana, D. (2018). *The polyvagal theory in therapy. Engaging the rhythm of regulation.* New York: W.W. Norton & Company.

Fisher, J. (1999). *The work of stabilization in trauma treatment.* Paper presented at The Trauma Center Lecture Series. https://janinafisher.com/pdfs/stabilize.pdf

Fisher, J. (2017). *Healing the fragmented selves of trauma survivors: Overcoming internal self-alienation.* Oxford: Routledge.

Gendlin, E.T. (1996). *Focusing-orientated psychotherapy: A manual of the experiential method.* New York: Guilford Press.

Gilbert, M., & Orlans, V. (2010). *Integrative therapy 100 key points techniques.* London: Routledge.

Goodchild, C. (2015). *The naked voice. Transform your life through the power of sound.* Berkeley, CA: North Atlantic Books.

Herman, J. (1992). *Trauma and recovery. The aftermath of violence -from domestic abuse to political terror.* New York: Basic Books.

Levine, P. (1997). *Waking the tiger: Healing trauma.* Berkeley, CA: North Atlantic Books.

Malchiodi, C. (2020). *Trauma and expressive arts therapy, brain, body and imagination in the healing process.* New York: Guilford Press.

Newham, P. (1998). *Therapeutic voicework. Principles and practice for the use of singing as a therapy.* London: Jessica Kingsley Publishers.

Ogden, P., & Fisher, J. (2015). *Sensorimotor psychotherapy: Interventions for trauma and attachment.* New York: W.W. Norton & Company

Steele, K., Boon, S., & Van der Hart, O. (2017). *Treating trauma-related dissociation: A practical, integrative approach.* New York: W.W. Norton & Company.

Peper, E., Pollock, W., Harvey, R., Yoshino, A., Dubenmier, J., & Anziani, M. (2019). Which quiets the mind more quickly and increases HRV: Toning or mindfulness? *NeuroRegulation.org,* 6 (3), 128–133. www.neuroregulation.org/issue/view/1553 DOI: 10.15540/nr.6.3.128

Porges, S. (2011). *The polyvagal theory: Neurophysiological foundations of emotions, attachment, communication, self-regulation.* New York: W.W. Norton & Company

Rappaport, L. (2009). *Focusing-orientated art therapy. Accessing the body's wisdom and creative intelligence.* London: Jessica Kingsley Publishers.

Rothschild, B. (2000). *The body remembers: The psychophysiology of trauma and trauma treatment.* New York: W.W. Norton & Company.

Schore, A.N. (2001). The effects of early relational trauma on right brain development, affect regulation, and infant mental health. *Infant Mental Health Journal,* 22, 201–269. www.researchgate.net/publication/237459576_The_Effects_of_Early_Relational_Trauma_on_Right_Brain_Development_Affect_Regulation_and_Infant_Mental_Health   DOI: 10.1002/1097-0355(200101/04)22:1<201::AID-IMHJ8>3.0.CO;2-9

Schore, A.N. (2003). *Affect dysregulation and disorders of the self.* New York: Norton & Company.

Siegel, D.J. (1999). *The developing mind: Toward a neurobiology of interpersonal experience.* New York: Guilford Press.

Storr, A. (1997). *Music and the Mind*. London: HarperCollins Publishers.

Van der Hart, O., Nijenhuis, E.R.S., & Steele, K. (2006). *The haunted self: Structural dissociation and the treatment of chronic traumatization*. New York: W.W. Norton & Company.

Van der Kolk, B.A. (2014). *The body keeps the score: Brain, mind, and body in the treatment of trauma*. New York: Viking Press.

Van der Kolk, B.A., & Fisler, R. (1995). Dissociation and the fragmentary nature of traumatic memories: Overview and exploratory study. *Journal of Traumatic Stress*, 8 (4), 505–525. https:/pubmed.ncbi.nlm.nih.gov/8564271/ DOI: 10.1002/jts.2490080402

Chapter 8

Working in partnership with service users experiencing anxiety, depression, and suicidal ideation in individual therapy, using the therapeutic relationship framework as a model for integration

Jude Smit

This chapter explores how a therapeutic approach can be developed in partnership with adults and young adults presenting with anxiety, depression, suicidal ideation, and trauma in hospital, Further/Higher Education, and private practice settings using the therapeutic relationship framework developed by Clarkson (2003) and Gilbert and Orlans (2011). I will highlight how Integrative Arts Psychotherapy can adapt, creatively and rigorously, to take account of the client's individual experiences and needs. The chapter further aims to demonstrate how this approach can support safe and ethical practice and how working in a trauma-informed way can allow space for what has remained hidden to come to light in a safe, contained, and timely way. By working integratively, the arts and visual narratives can aid the process of discovery and develop a shared understanding of clients' inner and outer worlds, using different art forms to deepen and enhance the client's engagement with creativity and imagination. Clients' reflections are included to honour the working partnership.

The work in context

An evidence-based framework, underpinned by theory and research into the treatment of anxiety and depression (Gilbert, 2007), supports my clinical thinking. This includes the impact of early relational trauma and related issues with intimacy, negative self-concept, and shame (Van der Kolk, 2014; Greenwood, 2011; Cundy, 2019; Jacoby, 2017). It provides insights into neuroscientific and neurobiological processes, the effects of unstable foundations, and how to practice safely and manage affect regulation and integration (Van der Kolk, 2014; Rothschild, 2021; Gerhart, 2015; Greenwood, 2011). In addition, it builds security by considering attachment dynamics in the therapeutic relationship (Holmes & Slade, 2018). When working with risk in suicidality, evidence-based practice into

DOI: 10.4324/9781003155676-12

suicide prevention (Pompili & Tatarelli, 2011) enables me to consider implications for therapy (Campbell & Hale, 2017) and the perspectives that support an integrated understanding of suicidal states of mind (O'Connor, 2021). By reading widely, I draw on the experience of others to review how the arts have supported them in their work (Case & Dalley, 2006; Schaverien, 1999) and also the efficacy of arts psychotherapy for anxiety, depression, suicidal ideation, and trauma in adults (Abbing, et al., 2018; Gilroy, 2006; Rothwell, 2008) and evidence that the use of the arts in therapy can affect change and improvement of symptomatology (Ciasca, et al., 2018).

It is clear from the literature that much of the work in attending to feelings of anxiety, depression, suicidal ideation, and trauma will require us to spend time in places that can feel very difficult for the client to visit. Exploring these might also trigger memories of events and experiences that have been traumatic or bring to life relational dynamics from past experiences with others in the therapeutic relationship. Many of these experiences are understood, thought about, and managed differently within cultural contexts. Therefore, it is important to be mindful of difference and to work collaboratively with clients to come to a shared understanding of the layers of complexity.

There can be many reasons why clients present with anxiety, depression, and suicidal ideation. I have seen unconscious material emerge in art making, revealing or containing trauma in subtle ways within the artwork. Working in a trauma-informed way allows me to hold in mind that to survive, there may be particular experiences that the psyche has needed to hide away. Contrary to some arguments that this way of working is reductive, experience has shown me that a trauma-informed approach does not close off or inhibit any possibilities. Pacing and grading the work together, whilst cultivating uncertainty and curiosity (Staemmler, 2009), allows space for clients to bring what they need to and provides the containment to be able to apply the "trauma brakes" (Rothschild, 2004), if necessary.

Considerations

I see part of my role as a container for unbearable experiences (Bion, 1984), with the capacity to hold the material with, and sometimes for, the client until it feels more bearable and manageable for the client to process. Sometimes, when there are no words for experiences, the arts enable unconscious processes to be brought into conscious awareness and reveal the felt sense of "the unthought known" (Bollas, 1989). I am open to "seeing" beyond what is shown and hold this for the client until they are ready to explore it together. One client reflected, *"When we have 'parked things' it has been really helpful, 'let's just leave that for now'. I have always been able to believe in that 'for now'"*. This way, together we can learn to recognise and stay within the client's window of tolerance (Siegel, 2015) and to hold challenging material within the framework of the six therapeutic relationships.

The stigma around suicide means that it remains a "whispered word" (Grollman, cited in Cholbi, 2011, p. 159). There is still much work that needs to be done to destigmatise and fear that talking about it openly will increase suicidal thoughts is a misconception. Research shows that open discussion can help reduce ideation and intent (Dazzi et al., 2014); the greater the fear of judgement and disempowerment, the less likely the individual will feel able to bring their authentic self. A client with lived experience expressed that *"People need to listen and understand how hard it is to reach out"*. To build a place of understanding, we need to learn from someone's lived experience, for the individual to feel not just listened to, but heard and validated. Therefore, I aim to provide a safe, contained environment where the client can bring themselves fully, without self-censoring. Working in partnership, we recognise and manage risk, projections, and relational patterns and explore potential new ways of being or relating.

From the start of our work together, my client and I think about their previous experiences of any power dynamics and how these might impact our therapeutic relationship. Clients' personal experiences of intersectionality and difference may have been painful and divisive. Therefore, holding in mind the representational layer of the relationship helps us to explore how I am seen. Identity is a significant part of the representational relationship and openly working with transference and projections can provide space to explore and share these feelings and perceptions.

I have found that being "real", present, and able to stay with difficult feelings and manage a range of affect, at times in its extreme, is an important part of the process, and for clients to know that our relationship will hold and survive ruptures. I actively create opportunities to work with the transference by empowering the client to bring projections and transferential feelings. A client described how working through these dynamics was transformative: *"Our sessions 'unpick' various uncomfortable situations and give me a better understanding of the patterns I've always got into"*.

I believe that we need to invite and welcome the transference and understand that projections are often driven by fear or hurt so that we can offer a reparative experience. I have been many things to many people in the transference: a parent, a sibling, a partner, a love object, and a former therapist. Being open to and meeting all these with acceptance, kindness, and empathy has enabled clients to bring their sadness, anger, and emerging feelings of attachment and love so that the energy can shift and they can internalise the "good object" of therapy (Kohut, 2014). At times I use creative adjustments – the arts, imagery, and metaphor – to mediate, hold, and bridge, deepening this process of understanding and connection, and once processed, move beyond the transference to the transpersonal.

An essential part of this process is an investment in my ongoing learning and reflection through the use of supervision. It enables me to ensure that I maintain safe, ethical, best practice, by actively and creatively engaging with the layers of complexity. I am hereby able to stay in contact and be fully present, whatever my clients bring, supporting us through the changing landscape of each individual's therapeutic journey and my own lifelong learning. Part of this work is my willingness to consider and own my potential part in the transference and representational relationship, by creating space to explore this both within the session and personally, through self-supervision and supervision.

Initial meetings

When meeting a new client and thinking together about our journey ahead, I use a metaphor to illustrate how I see this unfolding. We are in a car together; the client is in the driving seat and I am in the passenger seat with a map. We plan our route together and from time to time we make a stop to re-evaluate our journey, but I stress that the client remains the driver. I do not have an accelerator, the client is in control, and we go at a pace that feels manageable for them. The only dual control I have is a brake, as there may be times when I see something in our path that means we need to slow things down. To address any potential power differentials, I ask the client to tell me if at any point it feels like I am in the driving seat, as this is a helpful indicator for any possible transference reactions.

My wish is to truly know what life has been like for each individual and to build a working partnership where I think "with", not "for". The only way to truly know someone's experiences is for them to trust you and let you in so that you are able to experience and feel with them and through them. This image came to mind for my client:

> *You don't so much guide me down a path, as show me all of the paths that there are. It is like going on a hike together, I could say 'let's carry on down this path', you could show me there are another two and we go down whichever one I want to go down.*

As part of our first meeting, I carry out a comprehensive risk assessment so that we can work safely and I can grade interventions with risk in mind. The context, including presenting issues, setting, and referral type, is integral to thinking about and managing expectations. To work safely enough, sometimes clients require additional support structures to enable them to be in the world. This means that it can be more helpful for them to be held within a multidisciplinary team. I have been fortunate to work with some excellent teams where treatment and support have been considered holistically, for example, factoring in community support networks, having out-of-hours support available, and managing breaks. I adopt a co-created and collaborative approach, involving the client in this process to support them in building a sense of empowerment and agency so that we can think together about the most helpful approach to take. A client described their experience of this process: "*Working in partnership is really helpful for me because it gives me the freedom and control, I need to feel secure, while also helping me in times when I'm too overwhelmed to make decisions myself*".

After the session, I may use response art to capture some of the embodied richness and depth of the meeting and gain insights that imagery provides (Fish, 2017; Nash, 2020). I take time to think about and reflect on the six facets of the therapeutic relationship, focusing on each of these in response to the client and their unique lived experience. This enables me to look at how best to build a working alliance and to think about the challenges that therapy might bring for this individual – anticipating impasses, ruptures, and the experiences of breaks and endings – from the start of our work. I then formulate an initial treatment plan in partnership with my client, which we will review and revise regularly along the way. One client reflected that, *"Working in partnership is empowering"*.

Building a working/therapeutic alliance with clients who have experiences of anxiety, depression, and trauma

Working relationally and in partnership with clients, I believe that there are five elements integral to working practice: integrity, authenticity, transparency, empathy, and safety. I start all therapeutic relationships by meeting my client where they are without judgement or expectation, bringing myself to our sessions with warmth, openness, and a grounded, authentic presence that can start the process towards building trust and reparation. Clients who present with painful, traumatic experiences often arrive at the first session having had to survive in a hostile world, where trust has been broken. To build a robust working alliance, the client will need to feel confident that I can hold them and what they bring without judgement, but with patience, understanding, and empathy.

It is important to recognise that some clients have had little or no containment in their childhood or adult lives. Providing a secure, therapeutic framework with clear boundaries and mutual expectations is important, as this helps to create a consistent space that can come to be recognised as safe. One client explained how they experienced our relationship:

> *Trust, patience, understanding, honesty and open communication, meeting in the same neutral space each week, respect"* and noted: *"The high level of trust we've built up has allowed me to be more aware of what I'm feeling and to explore why I'm feeling that.*

The therapeutic alliance is fundamental to establishing and maintaining the relationship and it will support a client to stay in relationship, even when it feels difficult to be in therapy. With this in mind, I need to prepare the foundations by explaining that although therapy can be an empowering process of self-discovery, there may be times when it feels difficult and seems hard to persevere. In one of these discussions, my client really understood this. They helped me to know how best to support them at a time when trust is harder, or after a rupture, by explaining that for them, *"To be so honest with someone, you have to feel like you can do so on your own terms"*.

My client drew an image that captured their experience of the working alliance in therapy (Figure 8.1). While trapped in a dark and frightening place, filled with threat, our weekly therapy sessions provided a fragile lifeline.

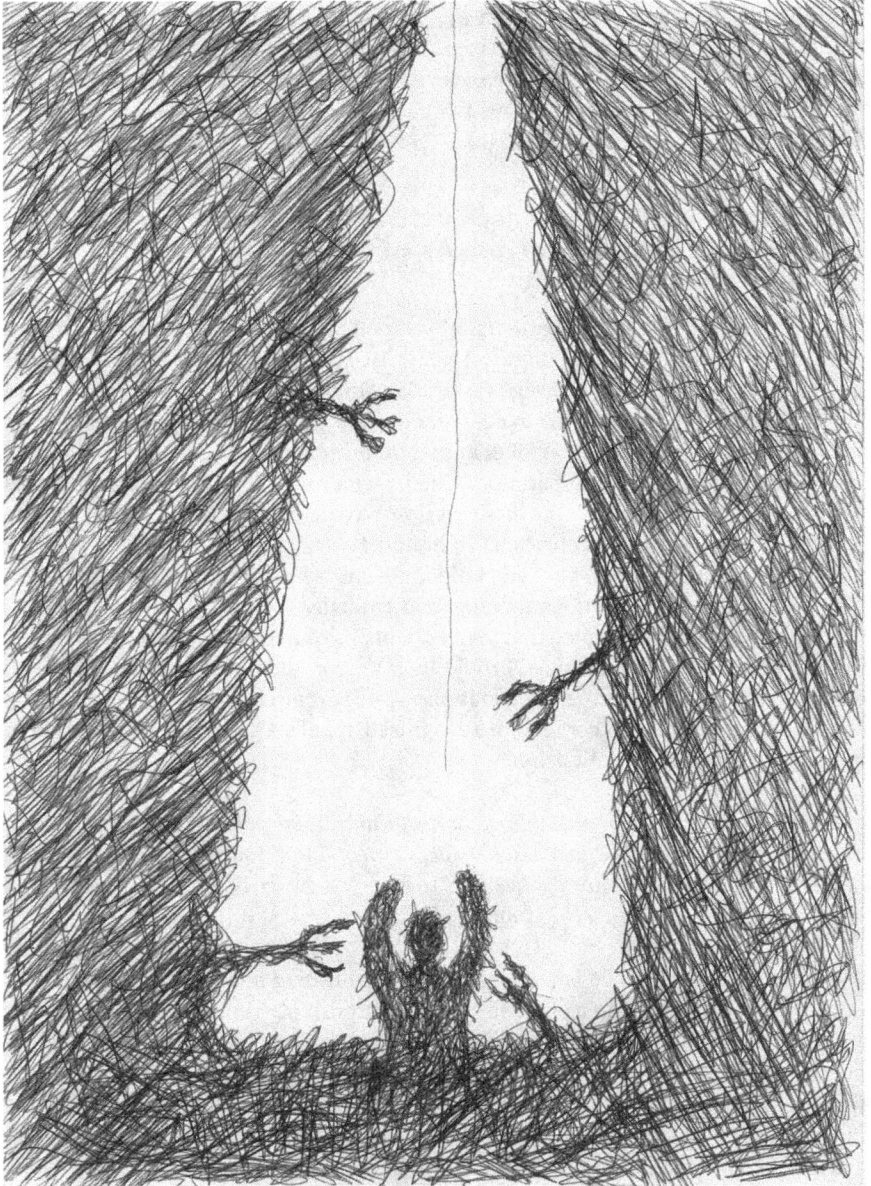

Figure 8.1 "Faint Hope (forever out of reach)"

Exploring the impact of lived experiences on the self

Depression and suicidal ideation can be *"very isolating, particularly at certain times"*. Part of the person-to-person relationship is normalising and validating the reality that sometimes each day is a challenge and it takes every effort to get up and face another day. One client described, *"Depression is anhedonia; apathy; not being able to see a future for myself"*. Using metaphor and imagery, another client was able to define their embodied experience: *"Depression is debilitating, it makes me feel like a lake that is slowly freezing over and becoming stiffer and stiffer with every second. It hurts and aches and makes me feel like I might die"*.

I have worked with people experiencing suicidal thoughts and behaviours for many years. I have found that they have often needed to develop and maintain a presented self in order to survive, having split off and internalised parts that have felt judged, hurt, rejected, and shamed. They are hiding a shadow self. This shadow self is made up of others' internalised voices that haunt and torment them, leading to fixed narratives about the self and a deep-rooted sense of shame. It becomes increasingly difficult to engage with the world, as the all-consuming anxiety, driven by rejection and never feeling good enough, reinforces a need to withdraw and hide.

When life seems unbearable and totally alone, someone can be left not knowing how to, or wanting to, live anymore. Suicidal ideation is "rarely simply allowed to be the human, individual experience that it is" (Murphy, 2017, p. 41). The stigma that remains means it becomes hidden away. It is held in the shadows of the self and with it, the reasons that led to a place of not knowing how to live. At these times, the robustness of the therapeutic alliance can be tested. One client expressed that *"It has often been the case that our work together is the only inter-action and connection I have with another person . . . it is hugely valuable in that respect to keep a little bit of feeling that I have a part in the world"*.

I have been referred long-term service users with depression, anxiety, and suicidal ideation who have been unhelpfully termed "treatment resistant" in the past. They describe having had decisions about their treatment made for them, contributing to an already ingrained belief that they have no voice and are powerless. These clients have been part of a healthcare system for many years and have lost hope and meaning, particularly where repeated cycles of anxiety and depression have led to withdrawal and disconnect. When meeting them for the first time, they have all expressed feeling misunderstood and alone, never having experienced the conditions that enabled them to work with and through some of the associated feelings and fears. A client expressed the impact of this: *"In the past I have struggled with many doctors and therapists, so it makes it really hard for me to start new therapeutic relationships, in fear of being abandoned"*. They described getting to the same point where they felt stuck many times, at which point the therapist would always refer on. Working in partnership, we have been able to identify that the perceived "resistance" is driven by fear, based on previous experience that the vulnerable self, the true self, will be rejected, hurt, or abused.

This leads to what I call an "uncomfortably comfortable" place where however painful, staying with what is known is preferable to the unknown.

The impact of childhood experiences on adult functioning is widely recognised (Casement, 1992; Kahn, 1991), and for many clients, negative childhood experiences of rupture have led to insecure attachments (Bowlby,1993). Unconscious fears and abandonment and the lack of "good enough" (Winnicott, 2005) parenting result in a child's inability to manage ruptures and fearing total annihilation (Klein and Mitchell, 1991). This primitive fear can challenge adult perceptions and cause difficulty with emotional regulation, resulting in a world filled with threat and insecurity. An individual's attachment style (Bowlby, 1993) therefore provides me with helpful information for understanding a client's ways of relating, both in therapy and how they experience the world. Early relational experiences or developmental deficits all affect a person's emotional regulation and create patterns and ways of being. To the unconscious, time is suspended, meaning that in certain circumstances, the client might experience the present as if they are, once again, a child. Therefore, when clients experience extremes of feeling in response to certain events in the here and now, I often ask what age they feel, as this can be a helpful indicator where things have become "stuck".

By staying with the "stuckness" and using the arts creatively, both exploring dreams and working with movement and the body helped to reveal the immense fear that had presented itself in early life. Unconsciously, remaining in this familiar, "uncomfortably comfortable" place had been preferable to the terror of the unknown. Moving between art forms within the session, the visual arts intuitively gave shape and colour to unexpressed feelings. Reflecting on what had been particularly helpful, the client explained how the integrative arts, together with trust in our relationship, provided the conditions that had previously been lacking: "When I have struggled to communicate, we have been able to try different things that you have suggested, an idea of taking on a pose that shows what I feel". Working together with the client to understand the relational dynamics gave permission for their emerging self to reveal itself and helped them to feel met. They noted: "Drawing on those very different ways of working means I never feel like there's nowhere I can go".

For clients to feel able to stay beyond the point when things become difficult, we first need to acknowledge and address any fears of abandonment. Clients need to know that neither they, nor their material, are "too much", but that what they bring to therapy are relatable, understandable human experiences. One client expressed that what they found particularly helpful about our therapeutic relationship was "Learning to build my own boundaries and not overstep them". They continued, "This time round I have been given complete control over what is talked about and worked on in therapy and it really helps me to feel reassured that I can say whatever I want".

I try to provide an environment where I can help clients recognise that sometimes life experience has meant that they needed to be strong for too long. It therefore takes real courage to show one's vulnerable self and to feel more able to bring the parts that have been hidden or shamed. When talking about the impact of shame, someone once told me that shame grows in unspoken places. This illustrates how trauma and shame can become so entwined with a person's sense of self that the person has literally been shamed into silence. When something has become part of identity, it needs to be treated with care and respect, as Yalom (2012, p. 151) states: "Never take away anything if you have nothing better to offer". A person's sense of self can be fragile, or the true self may have become so hidden that there is no real concept of having a sense of self at all, it feels lost, or even non-existent.

An emerging sense of self can feel threatening or frightening, as vulnerability has been avoided at all costs. At these times, I need to attend to the developmentally needed part of the relationship, so that the client can feel met and understood, to experience genuine care and compassion, without expectation or judgement. An essential part of processing attachment wounds is to acknowledge and recognise the grief that comes with these feelings, as grief does not only apply to the loss of someone who has died. I have witnessed grief for an unlived life, for a lost childhood, for a parent that never was, and for hopes and dreams that were abused and broken.

Using metaphor, I carefully weave in psychoeducation to help clients understand the pervasive nature and impact of shame that has become bound in with the self. I liken it to Japanese knotweed, which gets into the very fabric of a building, targeting the vulnerable places and threatening the building's foundations. It can lie dormant for up to 20 years and if you try to rip it out, it will regrow, each time weakening the structure further. It needs time and careful treatment, a planned approach so that the building remains secure and stable, whilst the knotweed is carefully removed. Some clients have used this metaphor as a starting point for art making. They have fed back that it has been a particularly helpful way to understand the impact on their life and how shame has been bound in with their depression, anxiety, suicidal ideation, and/or trauma.

One client explained how working creatively, with joint attention (Isserow, 2008) to this material, enabled them to slowly start building more self-compassion:

> Finally opening up about past traumas, and particularly the feelings and thoughts I have about them now, though distressing at times, has helped me start to come to terms with the fact that such things did happen. You have given me the opportunity to express feelings I have held for many years.

Their paintings depicted the visceral, raw reality of their lived experiences. Moving into sculpture enabled this to become more embodied, and finally the words that had gone unspoken made their way into poetry, giving a voice to all the pain and hurt. The reparative capacity of the therapeutic relationship can be transformational, as demonstrated by the client's recognition that "Our relationship is helping me to build a sense of self". Therapy enabled parts of the self that had been buried to emerge and experience acceptance and empathy (Kahn, 1991).

Therapy is able to serve as a transitional, transpersonal space, "inviting the lost heart of the self back into relationship" (Kalsched, 2013, p. 221). I believe that there is such beauty in vulnerability, but vulnerability needs to be respected and honoured, as this is where the true self can be met in creativity. The beauty of this process is experienced in the liminal spaces (Denham-Vaughan, 2018), meeting and connecting beyond the spoken, with all the pain, hurt, anger, and fear. For someone to know that I am here to hold this with them, completely accepting what is brought as lived experience, not as defining who they are. My client reflected, *"Knowing that you are always there and that there is no judgment, even if I were to sit silently through the whole session"*.

Conclusion

Working with clients who have experienced anxiety, depression, and suicidal ideation requires careful thought and a rigorous trauma-informed approach. I have found that the therapeutic relationship framework provides a useful model when working collaboratively and in partnership. Each of the layers of the relationship brings unique opportunities to explore and connect with our clients. Taking account of these from the start supports a therapist to plan creatively across the journey and the phases of therapy.

One of the reasons I decided to train and work as a therapist was due to the belief that by working in partnership, therapy has the capacity to be reparative and bring about change. Working with clients living with anxiety, depression, trauma, and suicidal ideation and behaviours in a range of different settings, I have come to understand that it is not always about achieving change. It is the process of honouring what is shared with total acceptance and sometimes climbing down into the pit to be with and stay alongside in the darkest places, when all feels hopeless. It is a real honour and privilege to be invited into the client's inner world and to know it more fully and deeply through the creative process.

As my client noted:

> *Isolation is that, without being able to connect I don't feel like I'm really existing, sometimes driven by not wanting to, to shy away from verification of my existence. Even at those times I manage to come to our sessions and you welcome me.*

References

Abbing, A., van Hooren, S., de Sonneville, L., Swaab, H., and Baars, E. (2018) The effectiveness of art therapy for anxiety in adults: A systematic review of randomised and non-randomised controlled trials. *PLOS One*, 13:12. DOI:10.1371/journal.pone.0208716

Bion, W. (1984) *Learning from experience*. Oxford: Routledge.

Bollas, C. (1989) *The shadow of the object: Psychoanalysis of the unthought known*. New York: Columbia University Press.

Bowlby, J. (1993) *The making and breaking of affectional bonds.* London: Routledge.

Campbell, D., and Hale, R. (2017) *Working in the dark.* Oxford: Routledge.

Case, C., and Dalley, T. (2006) *The handbook of art therapy.* East Sussex: Routledge.

Casement, P. (1992) *On learning from the patient.* London: Routledge.

Ciasca, E., Ferreira, R., Santana, C., Forlenza, O., do Santos, G., Brum, P., and Nunes, P. (2018) Art therapy as an adjuvant treatment for depression in elderly women: A randomised controlled trial. *Brazilian Journal of Psychiatry.* July–Sept 2018, 40:3, 256–263. DOI:10.1590/1516-4446-2017-2250

Cholbi, M. (2011) *Suicide: The philosophical dimensions.* Toronto, ON: Broadview Press.

Clarkson, P. (2003) *The therapeutic relationship.* New York: Wiley Publishing Company.

Cundy, L. (2019) *Attachment and the defence against intimacy: Understanding and working with avoidant attachment, self-hatred, and shame.* Oxford: Routledge.

Dazzi, T., Gribble, R., Wessley, S., and Fear, N. (2014) Does asking about suicide and related behaviours induce suicidal ideation? What is the evidence? *Journal of Psychological Medicine.* DOI:10.1017/s0033291714001299

Denham-Vaughan, S. (2018) At the threshold: Meditations on will, grace, and liminal space. In Chidiac, M. *Relational organisational Gestalt.* London: Routledge.

Fish, B. (2017) Arts-based supervision. In *Cultivating therapeutic insights through imagery.* Oxford: Routledge.

Gilbert, M. and Orlans, V. (2011) *Integrative therapy: 100 key points and techniques.* East Sussex: Routledge.

Gilbert, P. (2007) *Psychotherapy and counselling for depression.* London: Sage Publications Ltd.

Gilroy, A. (2006) *Art therapy, research and evidence-based practice.* London: Sage Publications Ltd.

Greenwood, H. (2011) Long term individual art psychotherapy. Art for art's sake: The effect of early relational trauma. *International Journal of Art Therapy*, 16:1, 41. DOI:1 0.1080/17454832.2011.570274

Gerhart, S. (2015) *Why love matters: How affection shapes a baby's brain.* East Sussex: Routledge.

Holmes, J., and Slade, A. (2018) *Attachment in therapeutic practice.* London: Sage Publications Ltd.

Isserow, J. (2008) Looking together: Joint attention in art therapy. *International Journal of Art Therapy*, 13:1, 34–42. DOI:10.1080/17454830802002894

Jacoby, M. (2017) *Shame and the origins of self-esteem: A Jungian approach.* Oxford: Routledge.

Kahn, M. (1991) *Between therapist and client.* New York: W.H. Freeman and Company.

Kalsched, D. (2013) *Trauma and the soul.* London and New York: Routledge Taylor and Francis Group.

Klein, M., and Mitchell, J. (1991) *The selected Melanie Klein.* London: Penguin.

Kohut, H. (2014) *The restoration of the self.* Chicago: University of Chicago Press.

Murphy, A. (2017) *Out of this world.* London: Karnac Books.

Nash, G. (2020) Response art in art therapy practice and research with a focus on reflect piece imagery. *International Journal of Art Therapy*, 25:1, 39–48. DOI:10.1080/17454 832.2019.1697307

O'Connor, R. (2021) *When it is darkest: Why people die by suicide and what we can do to prevent it.* London: Vermilion.

Pompili, M., and Tatarelli, R. (2011) *Evidence-based practice in suicidology*. Cambridge: Hogrefe Publishing.

Rothschild, B. (2004) Applying the brakes. *Psychotherapy Networker*.

Rothschild, B. (2021) *Revolutionising trauma treatment: Stabilisation, safety and nervous system balance*. New York: W.W. Norton & Company, Inc.

Rothwell, K. (2008) Lost in translation: Art psychotherapy with patients presenting suicidal states. *International Journal of Art Therapy*, 13:1, 2–12. DOI:10.1080/17454830802102314

Schaverien, J. (1999) *The revealing image: Analytical art psychotherapy in theory and practice*. London: Jessica Kingsley Publishers, Routledge.

Siegel, D. (2015) *The developing mind: How relationships and the brain interact to shape who we are*. New York: Guilford Press.

Staemmler, F. (2009) *Aggression, time and understanding: Contributions to the evolution of gestalt therapy*. New York: Routledge, Taylor and Francis.

Van der Kolk, B. (2014) *The body keeps the score: Mind, brain and body in the transformation of trauma*. London: Penguin Books.

Winnicott, D. (2005) *Playing and reality*. Oxford: Routledge.

Yalom, I. (2012) *Love's executioner and other tales of psychotherapy*. New York: Basic Books.

Chapter 9

Online integrative arts psychotherapy

Emma Cameron

Scratch, scratch, scratch . . . we're halfway through our Integrative Arts psycho-therapy session, and Sara's chalk pastels are rasping across the textured paper in vivid, energised flicks of powdery, fiery orange and scarlet. Repeated rhyth-mic strokes swoop upwards and outwards. Using both hands now, she frowns in concentration, her breathing heavy as she connects with the long-buried emotion that's been held in her body.

"I'm right here with you, Sara. Let's make lots of room for this feeling", I encourage her. "What does this anger want to say to him?"
"Just – Get away! Get away!"

With my support, Sara is exploring and feeling into this new experience of pro-cessing her anger and releasing its adaptive power.

Sara releases the pastels and smooths her palms across the paper. Using the same upwards and outwards motion she smudges the sharp marks. I'm sensing a shift in her affective state.

"And now . . . I wonder what's happening?"

Sara brings her gaze up, her expression now opening into a peaceful, focused calm.

"I'm feeling clearer . . . lighter . . . and really kind of strong, too . . . It's weird . . . Like, now I really feel like I know that I can do that. I can push him away. He can't define me!"

Sara and I look at one another. She takes a deep breath and exhales slowly; my own breath follows, in recognition of the powerful work we've been engaged in. This pause, this mutual gaze, feels full – almost sacred. We are present to one another, and to ourselves, at this moment, in service of Sara's healing.

And yet in this intense, powerful moment of therapeutic connectedness, Sara and I are physically 300 miles apart, for this is online integrative arts psychotherapy.

DOI: 10.4324/9781003155676-13

The Zoom platform enables us to connect digitally, whilst the therapeutic relationship and process underlie our ability to connect in spirit, in mind, in emotion, and – I would argue – even in body.

So how did we get to this point? What needed to happen in order for my client and I to work together so powerfully even though geographically we are so far apart? That's what this chapter seeks to explore. I hope that this discussion will help other therapists access information and strategies to develop their online work safely, ethically, and effectively.

The Case vignette describing online integrative arts psychotherapy work with client "Sara" is anonymized, and details have been changed to protect anonymity. Permission for publication of the case vignette and artwork has been given in writing.

Sara, a 31-year-old marketing professional, found her way to therapy after suffering from significant anxiety for several years. A blog post on my website had appeared in Sara's social media feed; a few days later, after reading more around the subject, she decided to email me. Many prospective clients have a preference for a therapist with an understanding of a particular aspect of identity (e.g., culture, race, sexuality, gender, age, body size, and neurodiversity); Sara had already been able to glean some of this information from my website before contacting me.

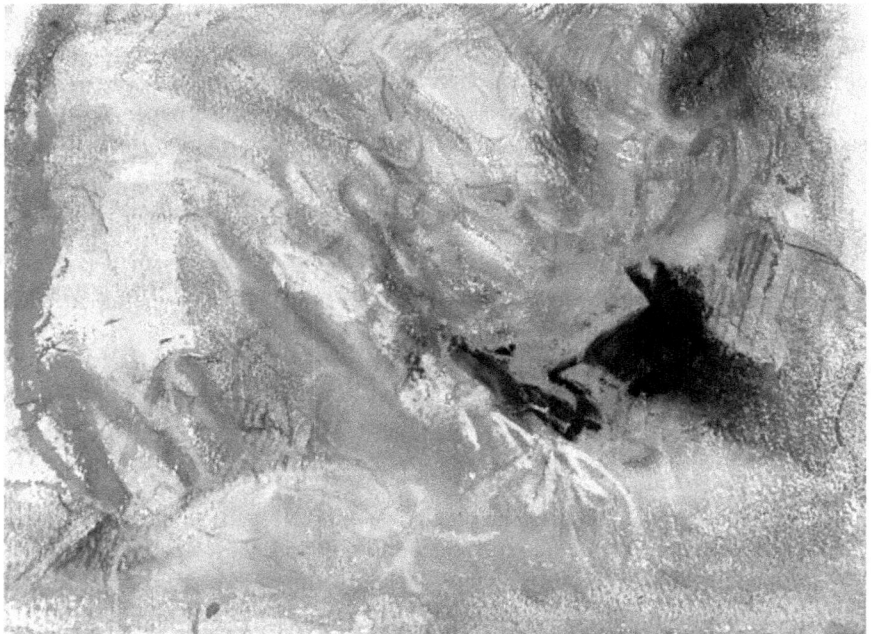

Figure 9.1 "Anger", by "Sara"

Suitability for online therapy

We organised an initial 20-minute phone call, to clarify what Sara was seeking help with and to discuss whether online integrative arts psychotherapy might be appropriate. I sought a brief outline of Sara's mental health history, and she identified her initial treatment goals. The assessment of a person's suitability for working online includes screening for psychosis or anything else that might make teletherapy unsafe or ineffective. Some situations may not necessarily preclude online treatment but may require third-party input (e.g., regular medical monitoring where someone has a restrictive eating disorder; basic technical support for persons with certain disabilities). A prospective client will need reasonably reliable internet access and a consistent, safe place where they can speak in privacy.

With safeguarding in mind, I checked whether Sara was currently living with a person who might pose a risk to her safety. (In situations of current domestic abuse, online therapy conducted from home is usually contra-indicated. A controlling and abusive partner could be listening in to a session, subjecting the client to harm afterwards.) Sara had a young daughter. It was important to establish that the child would safely be with another carer during our sessions, as Sara would need to be free to devote her attention to her own process.

Considering risk in online therapy

The online context poses additional risks, over and above those in traditional face-to-face (f2f) integrative arts psychotherapy. Therapists who are new to working online often worry about how they might manage, remotely, a client with suicidal ideation or who self-harms. Therapists are advised to think through how risk might be managed with a f2f client; then carefully consider whether any additional measures might be needed due to the client's location. A supervisor specifically trained in providing therapy and supervision online can be particularly helpful here (Stokes, 2018).

Zubala and Hackett's survey, "Online art therapy practice and client safety" (2020) posed the question "How do art therapists manage risk in online practice for themselves and for their clients?" (p. 162). The main concerns reflected in therapists' responses related to "online security/privacy" and "ethical considerations". Technical issues such as broadband connectivity were important concerns from a client's viewpoint, and the cost of equipment affected both clients and therapists. Security and confidentiality issues varied across the survey, with some therapists finding that they were less able to manage the risk of self-harm or suicidal ideation.

Where client data are held online, security is crucial. At the time of writing, I am using ProtonMail for email, Signal for texts and calls, and Zoom for video, because recent advice indicates these to be the most secure. However, recommendations are constantly subject to revision as technology continues to be developed. Other risks of online therapy, for client and therapist alike, include those that apply to anyone using computers and the internet (from hacking, phishing, viruses, and data leaks to more prosaic issues such as back pain, eye strain, and keyboard coffee spills).

Documentation

Having established that Sara and I might potentially be a "good fit", we agreed on a password for documentation. I emailed a form requesting contact details, date of birth, emergency contact, G.P., medications, and an outline of her mental health history. I also sent an information sheet, covering such topics as what to expect from online integrative arts psychotherapy, how to maximise confidentiality, some limits and risks of online therapy, payment procedures, and technology-related issues such as the necessity of keeping computer and applications updated, and tips for maximising bandwidth.

I noted where Sara would be having her sessions, and we agreed that if she were to have a session elsewhere, she would give me the address. This provides an additional layer of safety in the event of a health crisis or other emergency during a remote session. In the exceptional event of a client needing to have a session from a parked car, the 'What3Words' app can be used to provide a geographic location. I also sent Sara a GDPR document. This listed all the types of data that I would be collecting and keeping regarding her treatment, how I would maintain confidentiality, in what form data are held, why, and for how long. In the UK, organisations and individual private practitioners are required to maintain registration with the Information Commissioner's Office and must comply with data storage and handling regulations.

Starting a session

On the morning of our first session, I review the day ahead, emailing each client their Zoom link with its unique meeting number and password. A same-day reminder is a helpful *aide-memoire:* studies have shown that in comparison with f2f work, both clients and therapists may be more likely to forget online sessions (Russell, 2015). I check that I have tissues, glass of water, diary, pen, and notes to hand. I don't want to have to get up and move out of view partway through a session to fetch something. In f2f sessions, such interruptions feel minimal, but on screen, they can be disturbing to a client. Switching my mobile phone to silent, I check that any listening applications such as Siri, Echo, and Google Home have been disabled. This applies to phone, laptop, and any "smart" appliances nearby. On my laptop, I turn off notifications and to maximise bandwidth I quit the internet browser, email, and other applications. I also ensure that I won't be disturbed or overheard.

I log into Zoom a couple of minutes early and connect my earphones (with microphone) or headset. Without these, there can be a tendency to project one's voice in order to be heard, losing the softer vocal tones that help signal safety to the autonomic nervous system (Porges, 2011). Earphones also bring an extra layer of confidentiality: if anyone were to try and listen in from outside my room, they would not be able to hear my client.

Entering and leaving a session

It's our session time, but for a minute or two, there's no sign of Sara. I check my phone in case she has left a message. Having my mobile phone next to me, charged and switched on, means that we can message if necessary, and provides a backup in case my laptop encounters a problem. Clients' numbers are password-protected and stored under a code name on my devices. There are no messages, and soon Zoom informs me that Sara is in the "waiting room", so I let her in. This is our first moment of seeing each other's faces – a moment of surprise, curiosity, and some anticipatory anxiety. In an f2f session, some of the initial tension of this moment can be discharged through physical procedures such as removing the coat, arranging bags, and settling into seats. By contrast, arrival into the online setting can feel abrupt, and a client may feel anxious and hyper-vigilant. Naming and normalising this can help to regulate anxiety.

An f2f integrative arts psychotherapy session would typically involve a series of steps for a client: leaving their house, negotiating traffic and pedestrians; and on arrival ringing a doorbell or typing in a door code. The therapist might greet the client at the door, or in the waiting room, and they would walk together to the consulting room. This active, spatially complex process, typically spread out over an hour or so, is dramatically constricted when we meet online. In Sara's case, she would sometimes have to log out of a work meeting and then instantly enter her therapy session. Together we thought about what could help her to drop down from "business mode" into a more "right brain" way of being and relating. We found that a brief body scan at the start of a session, incorporating the breath and present-moment awareness, helped to ground and settle our nervous systems, so we could both fully "arrive" into the relational realm of therapy. Art making was also very helpful in this regard.

In f2f therapy, the setting contributes to a power imbalance. The therapist is familiar with the room and its contents, whereas a first-time client is presented with a new, perhaps daunting, environment. There's a lot to get used to: seating arrangements; smells; stray sounds from outside; all the arts materials; temperature of the room; and lighting. A client may have to contend with hints of others who have used the room before them: they may notice just-washed paintbrushes, warm seat cushions, or marks in the sandtray. By contrast, online therapy can afford the client more control and familiarity. Sara experienced a sense of agency and confidence due to being in her own space, appreciating "home comforts" such as comfy cushions and the warmth of her cat. She felt a sense of safety in knowing that she wouldn't have to face busy pavements straight after sessions when she was feeling undefended and vulnerable.

For a client like Sara whose job involves working online from home, having therapy in the same context risks a blurring of boundaries and potentially minimises the attention given to the therapeutic process between sessions. Straight after therapy, a client may be jolted back to returning their boss's urgent calls, managing bickering teenagers, or interacting with their spouse. Or, if their laptop is still open, a client might turn to social media to numb feelings and suppress thoughts after an emotionally intense session. I helped Sara think about how to protect her emotional space immediately before and after our meetings. She decided that she would try to take some space to journal, or just stand in her garden with a cup of tea for a few minutes as she let her thoughts and feelings settle.

Presence

In integrative arts psychotherapy, the therapeutic relationship is a primary meta-therapeutic factor (Norcross & Lambert, 2019), and we use the six-relationship framework to envisage this in its fullness (Gilbert & Orlans, 2010). The therapist's ability to be fully present (Siegel, 2012) with the client is key. This can be challenging enough face to face; working online throws up additional difficulties. How can we feel present with the client, and have them receive and experience our presence, when we are not even in the same room? Or when our computer suddenly informs us, "Your internet connection is unstable"? What about when there's a glitch and we miss part of a sentence; or when the screen is fuzzy and we can't quite see whether there's a tear in our client's eye, or pick up on subtle pencil marks or textures in their drawing? Geller (2020) specifically explores the issue of online therapeutic presence; this chapter aligns with many of her recommendations.

Gottlieb (2019, p. 136) describes online sessions as "therapy with a condom on", noting that sensory information may be dulled or unavailable, and it may feel harder to pick up on emotional resonance and energy. Therefore, therapists may need to be more proactive in style when working online. Sara soon got used to my frequently asking direct questions, such as "what are you noticing inside right now?" and "I'm wondering what it was like for you just now when I said x?"

Intentional amplification of the relational dimension can be very helpful when working online. Direct enquiries and comments that allude to the relationship and the contact boundary between therapist and client can build bonds and strengthen the therapeutic container. I was aware that such interventions can be challenging and need to be used with awareness and care; Sara, like most clients, had some difficulties tolerating closeness. Sometimes Sara's nervous system would begin to become hyper-, or hypo aroused. It is important to help a client stay just within their "window of tolerance" (Siegel, 1999) – the degree of nervous system arousal that allows for productive therapeutic work – so I would utilise grounding techniques when necessary.

In online therapy, it is easy for a client to withdraw or shut down, perhaps due to shame, distraction, or an avoidant attachment style; the lack of a shared physical space can contribute to this. When this happened with Sara, I found I could some-times gently invite her to reconnect with me through eye gaze, even if only for a moment, using a relational intervention such as "Could you take a peek at me right now? What do you see in my face?" When used judiciously, this could some-times help undo shame, loosen transference projections, and strengthen a sense of the reparative therapeutic relationship. The reparative relationship is one aspect of the six-relationship framework (Gilbert & Orlans, 2010) embedded in integrative arts psychotherapy.

I used other relationally charged interventions, such as "Can you feel me with you right now?" and "I'm right here, Sara", to undo Sara's aloneness (Fosha, 2021). Many therapists would hesitate to use these online, because of a literal interpretation of what it means to be 'with' someone. But in this technological age, I would argue that even when therapist and client are in completely different geographical places, it is indeed possible to be very much "with" one another in time, in awareness, and in emotional and neurobiological resonance.

Bringing in the body

Integrative arts psychotherapy involves paying attention to the body. Traumatic experience is held somatically (van der Kolk, 2015). The body is also used for grounding and for strengthening the capacity for dual awareness (Rothschild, 2010). Affects are body-based, and a client who is cut off from their somatic experience is restricted in their capacity to experience the relief and healing that comes from processing emotions to completion (Fosha, 2021). Yet the fundamen-tal experience of being two bodies in a room together, with its implicit "potential to kiss or kick" (Russell, 2015) is unavailable in online therapy. So how can we involve the body when we are working online, and not experience self and other as two disembodied sets of head and shoulders?

Integrative arts psychotherapy may have an advantage here over talk ther-apy. I encouraged Sara to pay attention to her sensory experience with the arts materials. Questions like "Ooh, what's it feel like to squeeze the play-dough like that?" and "I'm curious – is your paper rough or smooth?" helped her take in that I really wanted to feel into her experience. With my own equip-ment to hand, I would sometimes join Sara in exploring the materials; this helped create a sense of being physically connected despite working virtu-ally. The integrative arts psychotherapist can also make explicit that they value somatic information from the client. We can't rely on our own observation in the same way online as in f2f sessions, so instead of "I'm noticing your hands are clenched", I might enquire "I'm wondering what your hands are doing right now". Therapists sometimes worry that these questions will feel intrusive to the client, especially when used repeatedly, and to some clients, they might. However, very often clients will report, as Sara did, that being asked frequently about their somatic experience helps them internalise the ability to observe and be curious about themselves.

Advance preparation, and asking permission, can be helpful: "Part of the way I work is that I'll sometimes ask you what you're noticing in your body; will that be okay with you?" Early on, I accustomed Sara to somatic enquiry by offering a "menu" of examples of the kinds of things that she might notice and communicate, such as "butterflies" in the gut, clenched hands, a jiggling leg, or a knot in the throat (Ogden & Goldstein, 2020).

Miscommunications and glitches

Online therapy holds potential for misunderstandings, disconnections, and for a client to feel that they have been "missed". It is also easy for a session to be abruptly and prematurely ended, whether by client choice or through technological failure. This means that it is important for the online therapist to be clear and direct with a client. Sara and I regularly discussed what we would do in the event of connection issues (e.g., who would phone whom and on what number).

Many therapists consider that working online brings an increased sense of equality between therapist and client (Agar, 2020). Sara and I found that either of us could be subject to technical difficulties at times. When the inevitable glitches occurred, each needed to be forgiving of herself and of the other. Weinberg and Rolnick (2020) note that when technology is faulty or erratic, blame may be assigned – overtly or covertly, consciously or unconsciously – to the other person. This can be discussed with clients. Therapists should also be aware that when technology is functioning poorly, their frustration could lead to visible and/or audible expressions that are picked up by a client and may be experienced as an interpersonal rupture (Geller, 2020). Frequent checking-in and metatherapeutic processing as a session goes along can be helpful (Fosha, 2021). Sara got used to my asking questions such as "How did it land for you, when I said that?" and "What's it like for you now that we've had to turn our cameras off for a bit to improve the bandwidth?"

Handled well, a glitch can even help strengthen the therapeutic relationship: "What you're saying is really important, and I want to make sure I'm understanding. Would you mind repeating that last thing you said, because the sound cut out for a moment and I couldn't hear you properly". For Sara, who had never before experienced another person voicing a genuine desire to listen to her, moments like this were very impactful.

Use of the arts

Sara found it empowering to select and build her own collection of art materials. I offered some suggestions: basic art supplies, wet wipes, tissues, playdoh, and magazines for collage. Some therapists like to send a package by post, which can be particularly helpful for younger clients and those on a lower income.

Online, the therapist usually has limited sight of the art-making process. A client may choose to move their camera between their face and their art making, and the therapist may have to get used to asking the client if they would be willing to adjust their camera view. This requires a high degree of collaboration; when it works well it can be very beneficial for the therapeutic dyad. Sara opted to use her phone as a second camera, which she would direct down at the art-making activity. This was achieved by joining each session twice, once via her laptop and secondly (muted) with her phone.

Ogden and Goldstein (2020) encourage therapists to negotiate with each client about how to arrange themselves and one another so as to create a camera view that is bespoke and adaptive to the situation. Hands that are close to the camera will appear distorted in size, and expansive gestures may quickly slip out of the visual field, so there can be value in having a setup whereby each person can easily change position and distance in relation to the webcam. Sara liked using wireless headphones, which allowed her more freedom of movement.

During a session, the screen can be arranged so that the client and the therapist can view a completed image together and see each other at the same time. For example, a photo or screenshot of the artwork can be screen-shared by either party or the Zoom window re-sized so that faces can easily be seen. Technological advances open further options, such as digital sandtrays, and avatar-based virtual worlds such as ProReal Ltd (2021). Clients can be supported to use apps and programs for creating animations, collages, vision boards, digital books, and more. On-screen whiteboards on Zoom can allow client and therapist to collaborate in drawing activities.

Storage and Review of Artworks

Images created in art therapy can hold powerful emotional valence. Sara and I discussed how she would manage and store her physical artworks between sessions. I helped her to think about the potential reactions of family members, and she worked on setting boundaries that respected the therapeutic process and protected her privacy.

Zubala and Hackett's survey (2020) found that 47% of respondents felt that they were not able to offer a safe storage of the client's artwork (p. 165). I held digital images of Sara's work within a password-protected file, retained under a code name. For a review session, I created a PowerPoint file; Sara appreciated that I emailed her the file in advance so that she could screen-share at her preferred pace. For sharing images, password protection and the use of secure applications such as ProtonMail and Signal help to ensure confidentiality.

Silences and concealment

Whether online or f2f, a period of silence in a therapy session can hold a range of meanings and affects. Silences mediated by technology can present particular concerns, as it can be harder to identify what's going on, particularly when the broadband connection is imperfect. In online therapy, therapists may need to be more ready to break a silence themselves, perhaps by sharing their own process (e.g., "I'm noticing that my breathing's gone shallow – I wonder whether yours is doing the same?")

"[Online] the scope for projections and transference is inevitably greater than when we occupy the same physical space and breathe the same air" notes Cundy (2015, p. 102). Transference can show up in myriad forms. When therapy is digitally mediated, there is plenty of opportunity for transference to be expressed through the concealment of self or artwork from the therapist's view. Again, this presents opportunities for collaboration and discussion to help throw light on the interpersonal dynamic.

Clients may appreciate the control that the online setting offers. They can arrange themselves and/or their artwork to be seen or hidden according to what feels manageable and safe. Ogden and Goldstein (2020) offer an example of a client adaptively utilising the "mute" button, and moving off-camera, to explore an embodiment exercise, stomping and vocalising without triggering the feelings of exposure that might be experienced f2f.

The online disinhibition effect

The "online disinhibition effect" (Suler, 2004, 2016) is the phenomenon whereby actions and impulses that might normally be suppressed in face-to-face encounters are in the digital realm more likely to be expressed. "Trolling", hastily fired emails, and attacking comments on social media are examples. In online therapy, clients and therapists alike can find themselves affected by online disinhibition; this may be adaptive or maladaptive.

A client may be quicker to open up and show vulnerability online, compared to f2f. This can be beneficial for the therapeutic process. It also entails risks, as it may frighten a client, leading to them fleeing therapy prematurely. After one particular session, Sara experienced a shame reaction, feeling anxious that she might have revealed too much too soon. We found it helpful to slow the process down with frequent check-ins during a session, and I encouraged Sara to notice and communicate her experience as we went along.

Therapists, even seasoned ones, fall prey to the online disinhibition effect in a variety of guises. Many have found themselves doing something in an online session that they would never do face to face. This can range from the relatively benign (things like wearing slippers or sipping tea) to more concerning breaches. Examples include the over-sharing of personal information; slipping into a "chatty" mode of interaction; or repeated bending of the therapeutic frame with sessions extended, forgotten, or frequently rescheduled. Therapists are encouraged to stay actively curious about how the online disinhibition effect may be showing up clinically (Weitz, 2014).

Most integrative arts psychotherapists moved their work online during the pandemic lockdowns of 2020–2021, and many are continuing to make use of this option, at least in part. The Zubala and Hackett survey (2020) considers art therapists' adaptation to online service provision, noting that a majority will continue working online beyond the immediate impact of the pandemic. Whether we work online routinely or only occasionally, as professionals we have a responsibility to keep updating our knowledge and skills around the relevant technology (Pennington et al., 2020).

Conclusion

Compared to f2f, online integrative arts psychotherapy involves additional layers of complexity. As therapists, we need to pay attention to all of these layers. There are practical issues such as how to manage tech equipment; clinical choice points such as when and how to intervene when a client disappears from view; extra demands on the client with regard to holding the space, accessing arts materials, and storing images; limits on sensory experience, movement, and physicality; and new psychological aspects to consider, such as the online disinhibition effect.

The integrative arts psychotherapist works to engage the client, helping them deepen awareness and connect with their feelings through the experience of a meaningful therapeutic relationship and through the creative process. When this work takes place online, it is done in a context in which themes around disconnection and concealment are integral and unavoidable, whether these occur through psychological processes or through the "third party" of technology. Therapists may even notice apparent parallel processes at times, whereby psychotherapeutic themes appear to manifest via technological procedures and machinery.

In digitally mediated therapy, we are constantly reminded of the dialectic between presence and absence, connection and disconnection, openness and concealment, and flow and interruption. The challenge of conducting integrative arts psychotherapy is magnified and expanded when we take our work online; for clients like Sara, and for myself as her therapist, the rewards can be enormous.

References

Agar, G. (2020). The clinic offers no advantage over the screen, for relationship is everything: Video therapy and its dynamics. In: Weinberg, H. & Rolnick, A. (Eds.) *Theory and practice of online therapy: Internet-delivered interventions for individuals, groups, families and organisations.* 66–78. New York: Routledge.

Cundy, L. (2015). *Love in the age of the internet: Attachment in the digital era.* London: Karnac.

Fosha, D. (Ed.) (2021). *Undoing aloneness & the transformation of suffering into flourishing: AEDP 2.0.* Washington, DC: American Psychological Association.

Geller, S. M. (2020). Cultivating online therapeutic presence: Strengthening therapeutic relationships in teletherapy sessions. *Counselling Psychology Quarterly.* Available at: https://doi.org/10.1080/09515070.2020.1787348

Gilbert, M. & Orlans, V. (2010). *Integrative therapy: 100 key points and techniques.* London: Routledge.

Gottlieb, L. (2019). *Maybe you should talk to someone: A therapist, her therapist, and our lives revealed.* London: Scribe.

Norcross, J. C. & Lambert, M. J. (Eds.) (2019). *Psychotherapy relationships that work: Volume 1: Evidence-based therapist contributions.* Oxford: Oxford University Press.

Ogden, P. & Goldstein, B. (2020). Sensorimotor psychotherapy from a distance: Engaging the body, creating presence, and building relationship in videoconferencing. In: Weinberg, H. & Rolnick, A. (Eds.) *Theory and practice of online therapy: Internet-delivered interventions for individuals, families, groups, and organizations.* 47–65. New York: Routledge.

Pennington, M., Patton, R. & Katafiasz, H. (2020). Cybersupervision in psychotherapy. In: Weinberg, H. & Rolnick, A. (Eds.) *Theory and practice of online therapy: Internet-delivered interventions for individuals, families, groups, and organizations.* 79–95. New York: Routledge.

Porges, S. W. (2011). *The polyvagal theory: Neurophysiological foundations of emotions, attachment, communication, and self-regulation.* New York: W.W. Norton.

ProReal Ltd. (2021). *ProReal (version 3.7).* Digital application. Available at: https://proreal.world

Rothschild, B. (2010). *Eight keys to safe trauma recovery.* New York: W.W. Norton.

Russell, G. I. (2015). *Screen relations: The limits of computer-mediated psychoanalysis and psychotherapy.* London: Karnac.

Siegel, D. J. (1999). *Towards an interpersonal neurobiology of the developing mind: Attachment relationships, "Mindsight", and neural integration.* Available at: www.glasgow.gov.uk/CHttpHandler.ashx?id=17465&p=0

Siegel, D. J. (2012). *The developing mind: How relationships and the brain interact to shape who we are.* New York: Guilford Press.

Stokes, A. (Ed.) (2018). *Online supervision: A handbook for practitioners.* London: Routledge.

Suler, J. R. (2004). The online disinhibition effect. *CyberPsychology and Behaviour,* 7 (1), 321–326. Available at: www.academia.edu/3658367/The_online_disinhibition_effect

Suler, J. R. (2016). *Psychology of the digital age: Humans become electric.* Cambridge: Cambridge University Press.

Van der Kolk, B. (2015). *The body keeps the score: Brain, mind, and body in the healing of trauma.* New York: Penguin.

Weinberg, H. & Rolnick, A. (Eds.) (2020). *Theory and practice of online therapy: Internet-delivered interventions for individuals, families, groups, and organizations.* New York: Routledge.

Weitz, P. (Ed.) (2014). *Psychotherapy 2.0: Where psychotherapy and technology meet.* London: Karnac.

Zubala, A. & Hackett, S. (2020). Online Art therapy practice and client safety: A UK-wide survey in times of COVID-19. *International Journal of Art Therapy,* 25 (4), 161–171. Available at: www.tandfonline.com/doi/full/10.1080/17454832.2020.1845221

Part IV

Creative integration in practice – working with groups

Chapter 10

Self-reflective groups in action

Working with difference, politics, and the creative arts as a bridge for connection and taking up space

Anthea Benjamin

Introduction

In this chapter, I will explore the ways in which our understandings of ourselves and others are fundamentally shaped by the world we live in and the experiences we are exposed to. I am a black woman who has been facilitating personal development groups for over ten years. The re-emergence of issues about the misuse of power and privilege arising from events such as Grenfell, Black Lives Matter, and COVID-19 forcibly reminds us as a profession of the need to engage with issues of social justice that are directly encountered by our trainees, our clients, and ourselves. As a Group Analyst, I hold the individual's personal lived experience, their internal psychic world, and the socio-political context as being interconnected and all of equal importance. Art therapy has the potential to enhance the process of truly recognising ourselves and the world we live in, opening new ways of communication and social learning. This chapter explores some of the change processes that can take place in these group settings to address issues arising from intersectional identities and the power relations that are prevalent throughout society. 'Every personal development group member is faced with the challenge of learning to relate in a meaningful manner, to communicate at depth, to change and to grow. And to facilitate these processes in the client' (Rose, 2008).

Exploring the fullness of our identities

Personal development groups are a core feature in most psychotherapy and counselling trainings. The purpose of these groups is to fine-tune "self as instrument" (McWilliams, 2004). Art therapy offers a transitional space in which transference onto art materials, as well as onto group members, can take place (Winnicott, 1971). Through creative opportunities for symbolising their own feelings, beliefs, and value systems, students come to understand themselves and the communities they will work within. Art therapists often express the idea of the "arts as healing" (Levine, 1988) which is well meaning but does not adequately address dynamics and power relations. My lived experience has taught me to examine power

DOI: 10.4324/9781003155676-15

relations from an intersectional perspective considering poverty, racism, classism, sexism, homophobia, and other forms of social oppression (Talwar, 2019).

Personal development groups are closed and often non-directive and aim to reflect on interactions created through transformational experience (Johns, 1996). Beginning trainees are likely to have different levels of understanding about the various facets of their identities. This can lead to uneasiness with this type of learning approach (Anderson & Price, 2001). Drawing from the concepts of group interactive art therapy, using image-making can increase learning opportunities as it can enable the containment of powerful feelings (Waller, 2015). Personal development groups can use directive and non-directive methods in structuring the group's time, which include a balance of time spent talking and image-making in order to create a developmental space (McNeilly, 2006).

Group facilitators are repeatedly faced with complex choices about what to give time to, whom to give space to, and how to attend to interactions between members whilst creating space for the group to reflect on the interplay of personal, social, and political dynamics taking place. Bowlby (1988) illustrated the importance of a secure base for the developing infant; Foulkes (1964) sees the group as a maternal womb-like space. As group members communicate, they create a web of communication, which becomes a containing force for ongoing processes. The group facilitator's role is in supporting members in creating a safe enough space to explore, but not too safe to prevent growth through challenge. Encounter groups like these enable students to learn under pressure, build self-esteem, and strengthen the ego (Freud, 1960).

Levine (1992, 15) states, "The task of therapy is not to eliminate suffering but to give voice to it, to find a form in which it can be expressed". As a facilitator, I support members to reflect on differences between themselves and to find a shared language. Finding the right language to explore power, privilege, and positioning can be a minefield because of the limited language available to support discussions that are simultaneously inclusive and sensitive to the varied ways in which individuals identify. I will describe issues of power relations and will also use the term minority, although I recognise that in some cases, those categorised by the term minorities can in fact constitute most of the overall world population (Tatum, 1997).

Where do we start?

One of the ways I encourage groups to start the process of thinking about identity is through making images to introduce themselves. This can be through the use of miniatures, sandtray work, painting, clay, art, or any medium that they can make use of within the group setting. In my groups, I tend to have an extensive art tray available that members can use. When image-making takes place, group members either spread out individually or sit in small groups creating art to reflect themselves in meaningful ways. Their art will reflect the different identities such as culture, race, sexuality, ableism, age, gender, and any other social identities.

I do not work with a timetable, so it can be that the group is not always in agreement about when they want to make art. Members can sometimes be split, with some of the group wanting to stay with dialogue and other members wanting to move into using image-making. I try to allow the group to negotiate this without having to agree all the time, which is another way of modelling how groups can stay with and work with differences. This process often generates a sense of aliveness, which can lead to frustration when they have a preconceived way of how the group needs to work. When they can accept the group dynamics and what emerges in this process, members can bring different aspects of themself using the arts (Levine, 1992). For others, it can feel like a struggle; nonetheless, this process is just as important as it enables them to start to come to know themselves in a different way.

We are all subject to the subliminal messages we receive throughout society about power. When they are not interrogated, these messages often go on to significantly influence our thinking and experience of ourselves in the world. The personal development group enables members to do this investigation collectively (Lennie, 2007). After the group has completed making images, I ask them to introduce themselves to the group, using their art, naming their intersectional identities, and the language they use to describe themselves. This process is often immensely powerful. It provides a way for members to bring more of themselves into the group setting. I often have feedback that the group members find out so much more about each other and in more depth, this way. In addition, people find themselves more able to name their differences in relation to class, race, sexuality, etc. The work of the group is to manage the shame around public and private self-dynamics being brought to awareness so that the group can have the opportunity to learn from each other.

One of the common themes that often emerge from white members of the group is to believe that they have no culture, or they focus on a shame narrative about colonialism. These processes need to be honoured. It is also important to challenge these members to reflect in more depth on the wholeness of their cultures and not to stay stuck in a defensive response that can keep them from fully integrating aspects of their identity. When two contrasting aspects of the self-appear, I ask group members to check in and see if they need to have another image to hold the polarities of those parts of their identity. I will give them the opportunity to think about integration if this is something they want to do, or I stay with thinking about how they hold the aspects separately.

At each meeting, the group will start with talking, and then as themes emerge, we explore whether making art might be useful to deepen the process. Sometimes the group might want to start working with art forms, so that at the end of that process, we reflect on and speak about what has emerged from the images. My rule of thumb is to make sure there is at least 30–45 minutes within a 90-minute group session to process image making at the end of the group and, where relevant, to link this to the relationships within the group. Group members stay on for a bit of extra time to tidy up the group space, before leaving the session. This can include an intentional process of unmaking images or of returning (depositing) the art materials.

As time goes on . . .

Over time in the personal development group as topics surface, students bring in their experiences of their own lived social context. I encourage the group to take time to stay with these incidents and to think about how that positions them. This can be a very liberating and/or shaming experience, as it means members must name their position in the world, their prejudices, and stay with the reality of what this might mean and feel like. This process can enable students both to reflect further on their own identities and to reflect on how they read artwork, images, emotions, and experiences through an intersectional lens. This can empower students to be able to interrogate their own worldview and be more attuned to the impact of "otherness". Awareness about "positionality" (Madison, 2012) is key for art therapists in understanding how unconscious bias impacts how we facilitate art and see art in clinical practice. McNiff (1998) comments, 'creativity cannot flourish and reach its deepest potential without the participation of its demons as well as its angels'. The personal development groups create a transitional space (Winnicott, 1971) that can hold these polarities.

Using members' disclosures of personal experience in personal development groups can be helpful in unpacking members' values and positionality. In most groups, there will be some form of sub-grouping. It is helpful for this to be named in some way and to explore what is held in this grouping. I have found that this process can be facilitated through the arts, as a sub-grouping image can help members to explore their positions in the sub-groups and with each other. A challenge can arise if some members find themselves alone and not part of a group. However, this is useful for the group to take up and make sense of together. Group members then bring these images together to create a constellation of how they feel they are as a whole year group. This can tease out any unspoken dynamics and power dynamics within the groups and between members. Sometimes this can lead to the group wanting to create individual images of self, using the arts to consider how they would like to be in the group. This can be a beneficial way of discovering how members can experiment with roles in the group and beyond.

Rivalry, envy, and jealousy will often be present in any group since unconscious family dynamics and early infantile feelings get stimulated. These dynamics and feelings are amplified by the experience of being in a deskilled position by virtue of training and by the deep disturbance and trauma associated with experiences of deprivation and discrimination. Facilitators need to encourage the group to deal with their rivalry and to interrogate the impulse to create a hierarchy of oppression. Rivalry in groups normally revolves around competition for the facilitator's attention or rivalry between specific group members. Containment of these processes using image-making can enable the group to name and make sense of these dynamics and prevent this tipping into destructive processes. When these undercurrents occur in the group, I ask the group to share metaphors or images of their associations with these feelings in their bodies and link this to the process. There can be a "flight" reaction to move into art making to escape from these feelings, but I try to get them to stay with the feelings and to learn over time when art making is a deepening process or a form of avoidance. The use of imagery becomes a vehicle to help members to explore these powerful primitive processes and unwanted parts of themselves.

In one group, two group members explored their images of rivalry and named each other as the person they felt most rivalrous of in the group. They talked about the need to speak after each other or to contradict each other, often being pulled into this dynamic impulsively. They talked about this being particularly amplified in the personal development group, although they were aware of it in other aspects of their training too. As they talked to each other they expressed how nervous and awful they felt about the need to pull each other down, also the paradoxical relief and shame at naming this. The whole group was transfixed, as they watched them unpack their process. I supported them to think about this process and what it might be about each other, which seemed to urge them into this dynamic. I suggested that they think about what was similar between them and what might be different? They shared that they felt similar in their outspokenness and their need to be right. They then compared their differences, in terms of class – one went to boarding school, the other went to a state school, one lived a settled middle-class life with a wealthy partner, the other was a lesbian single mother working freelance. They went on to reveal several assumptions they had made about each other, including assumptions they had made about how they each felt about the other.

As this developed, the wider group remained silent. I wondered about "pairing" (Bion, 1959), a defence mechanism where the work of the group is held by two members. I then considered that this might reflect something for the group-as-a-whole. Reluctantly group members started to own their own rivalries, mostly towards the two group members who started this process. I challenged them to think about where else the rivalry was located and suggested they come up with their own imagery for this, as naming it directly seemed to feel too difficult. This opened the dialogue even more, as members felt contained by the imagery and could risk sharing their rivalry with other group members. The theme then turned to inferiority and a shared fear of not being "good enough". This linked to the deeper issues of their social positioning and personal histories about belonging, having space, and being seen. For example, one member disclosed she had grown up in poverty and had learned to take up as little space as possible, so as not to be a burden. She could see how this played out in the group and was amplified by her sense of the profession being a middle-class arena, in which she felt there was no space for her.

There are many ways to explore these themes without imposing them on the group. I tend to track themes as they arise, becoming curious about what is in the group dynamic, noticing what we are and are not engaging with, and wondering why? I also encourage members to reflect on what may be taking place in their bodies. This can be in the form of a body scan, noticing how they feel in their bodies and encouraging them to name that or to use an image to represent that sensation or feeling. This can then be considered as a group feeling, which the group can play with to begin to make some sense of the complexity of what might be present in the group field. We know that many people have learnt to hold the body as an object separate from self, in the same way, the internal world has been split off from the socio-political domain. The nature of socio-political violence, which operates throughout society, is in "othered" members and this is often located within the body. By building stamina to tolerate difficult feeling states in groups, members can understand how these intergenerational forms of trauma echo in the clinical work and be better equipped to manage.

Grappling with representation

One of the themes that also arise in personal development groups is about the lack of diversity within therapy training and how this is reinforced throughout teaching institutions (McKenzie-Mavinga, 2005). Members who have entered training from a different socio-economic class positioning may often find themselves feeling that they don't fit in. Talking about class and power differentials often induces guilt and shame in the group and, either consciously or unconsciously, there is a push to shut down the thinking (Bion, 1959). This can play out with members of marginalised groups taking on a role for the group. Foulkes (1964) describes his concept, the 'location of disturbance' as a psychological disturbance that takes place *between people* that can never really be confined to one person. The "location of disturbance" is a way of understanding how an individual can become a recipient of unconscious projections which reflect a wider group dynamic that is a blind spot for that wider group. The concept of the "location of disturbance" is important in helping groups to understand the projective scapegoating dynamic through conscious and unconscious processes taking place both in groups and throughout society.

Robin DiAngelo (2018) writes about "white fragility" a defence mechanism that occurs when race is discussed in groups. This results in explicit expressions of anger, fear, crying, defensiveness, or guilt. This type of white fragility is likely to occur in mixed-race groups when white members are challenged about their unconscious bias, particularly when people of colour speak about racism. They may ultimately be experienced by others as aggressive, which needs to be challenged and made sense of as a dynamic taking place both in the group and in the wider world context.

A similar defensive mechanism can be used by members of marginalised groups, who habitually create sub-groupings of safety that I will refer to as "shielding". These sub-groups can tend to remain invisible or silenced, due to their lived experiences of not being heard or having their experiences discounted or minimised. When facilitators do not explore these dynamics, they are complicit in maintaining the status quo. By supporting group members to expand their ability to stay with the discomfort of these conversations, the space can open up for more marginalised experiences to be heard. The fear for many marginalised groups is the re-enactment of unconscious bias in the group, which goes unnoticed and then leads to re-traumatisation. The work of the facilitator is to track these processes and any enactments that are likely to take place, such as defensive resistance of any subgroup and bringing awareness to these repetitions. Often what is missed for these members is their experience of internalised racism, homophobia, etc. These experiences are hard to address within groups settings, where the general membership is unable to address their own unconscious bias. There is often shame attached to these experiences and there needs to be a sense of safety in place to be able to address these patterns. Facilitators need to be sensitive to this and to support the group to hold these themes with compassion and, where needed, to challenge the group to face this.

An essential part of this process for a group facilitator is the ability to attend to the complexity of managing subgroup dynamics and maintain the cohesion of the group as a whole (Foulkes, 1964). It is important not only to find the balance that can enable all voices to have space but also to catch unconscious group re-enactments. For example, when one group member engages another member on the topic of the whole group's inability to tackle social justice issues, very quickly a split emerges in the group. Binary black and white thinking appears and there is a tendency to go into a paranoid–schizoid split, which focuses on who is right and who is wrong. The work in this moment is to slow the group down, keep group members thinking, and track bodily activations within the group. The use of the arts encourages mentalisation (Moore & Marder, 2020). It is an immensely help-ful tool in supporting group members to reflect on mental states, to recover their thinking, and to link this process to the wider world context. This was particularly true when I was running groups at the height of the Brexit debate. Members who felt unwelcome in this country talked in depth about feeling displaced and unsafe. There was a group urge to dismiss this and to create a narrative of "we're not like this". I asked the group to go into image-making to reflect on safety and belonging as the theme that appeared to be emerging in the group, in order to support mem-bers to make sense of their feelings. What struck me was how the use of tactile arts materials seemed to act as a tool for emotional regulation. On their return, they could reflect more about their feelings. Members who went into defensive guilt seemed also to have more capacity to stay with the real feelings of despair and hopelessness. The arts seemed to create more stamina and deepen the feeling states within the group. Over time members were able to name their own preju-dices about foreigners, including members who identified as foreigners. We were then able to explore the dynamics of "stranger" and 'othering' as a dynamic in the world, within the group and within themselves.

Putting things into words

Generally, in personal development groups, a facilitator will raise the topic of power relations and have a brief discussion about this – simply putting the topic on the agenda, so it can be returned to as needed. In my view there is a need to keep the topic in awareness in the group, to enable frequent conversations on these topics that may help to develop personal reflections over time (Eastwood, 2021). The ability of the group to engage in these conversations will develop, due to the group members' increased level of trust in the facilitator and members' understanding of his, her and their own racial/ethnic, gender, class, and other identity. Therefore, sensitivity to the timing and pace of these conversations, over the course of the personal development group, is important. There are clearly no universal rules for how and when to have these conversations, the important thing is that they take place.

The importance of psychoeducation in enabling students to see projective processes in action can help them to identify both their own blind spots, as well as group-related phenomena that take place throughout society. This approach requires members to make use of each other. They learn to take risks through their unfolding in-group interactions, which provides group members with valuable insights into how their behaviour can affect others. In time these insights can be transferred to relationships outside of the group, as well as to clinical practice.

At times, group facilitators may intentionally choose to disclose their own reactions to specific dynamics taking place within the group, for example, "I am feeling a huge sense of anxiety and difficulty engaging with this subject and I am wondering how others are feeling? This could also include naming what is not being engaged with, "*I am wondering what is not being said as I have a strong sense of avoidance taking place right now? Am I the only one feeling this way?*" In instances where conflict emerges, whether this is defensive or silencing of difference, it is important for the group facilitators to simultaneously acknowledge the validity of all group members' emotions and to identify ways in which these responses avoid important conversations about social justice and equality.

Holding the tension

As part of this process group facilitators will also experience their own instances of discomfort or feeling intimidated about how to respond to conflict arising from defensiveness or "shielding". Heightened emotions stemming from conflict about differences within a group are often powerful and explosive. At these times, it is important for facilitators to be aware when a group member may be avoiding a charged topic due to their discomfort. Group leaders must also be careful not to try to interrupt important group processes prematurely, to save the group by using interpretations aimed at making the process 'okay'. This is where ongoing work for facilitators is needed to address their own unconscious biases and to not become complicit with the unconscious avoidance of these themes within groups. This will be informed by the facilitators' ability to monitor their own responses to intense periods in the group and to see these as important data for what group members may also be experiencing. This is also key for facilitators, as they are also subject to these protective mechanisms. I have found this way of working exciting and challenging. As a facilitator, it means that you may be called out about your own unconscious bias, but this is a great way of modelling leadership with vulnerability and transparency (Brown, 2015). Considering the worldwide call for more inclusive practice, I find this way of working a helpful way for us all working together to ensure we hold each other accountable yet supported.

Conclusion

Creative arts therapists are skilled at supporting clients to explore their internal world. Intersectionality gives us a framework to support therapists to engage with their unconscious bias and responsibility to understand the principles of power, privilege, and positioning. It is important that we are all self-reflective and understand how our own lived experience can position us and give us a too specific lens with which to view image-making and group work.

As creative arts therapists, given that we are a predominantly white, heterosexual, and able-bodied profession, we each need to work actively to increase awareness of our own bias. For therapists to be effective at addressing the societal influences that negatively impact the mental health of marginalised groups, they need to be engaged with and acknowledge these power differentials and attempt to bring about social change alongside their clients. I am not suggesting that therapists need to be activists within their practice. That said, to meet the multicultural needs of clients we need to be able to hold their world view in mind, to fully understand a client's experience and positioning within society. In my view, personal development groups offer a unique and valuable opportunity to address this in a meaningful way within psychotherapy and counselling trainings.

References

Anderson, R. D., and Price, G. E. (2001) "Experiential groups in counsellor education: Student attitudes and instructor participation." *Counselling Education and Supervision* 41(2): 111–119.

Bion, W. R. (1959) "Attacks on linking." *International Journal of Psycho-Analysis* 40: 308–315.

Bowlby, J. (1988) *A secure base*. Abingdon: Routledge.

Brown, B. (2015) *Daring greatly: How the courage to be vulnerable transforms the way we live, love, parent, and lead*. London: Penguin.

Eastwood, C. (2021) White privilege and art therapy in the UK: Are we doing the work? *International Journal of Art Therapy* 26(3): 75–83. DOI:10.1080/17454832.2020.1856159

DiAngelo, R. (2018) *White fragility: Why it's so hard for White people to talk about racism*. Boston: Beacon Press.

Foulkes, S. H. (1964) *A memorandum on group therapy*. Oxford: British Military Memorandum, ADM.

Freud, S. (1960) *The ego and the id*, J. Strachey (Ed.). New York: WW Norton and Co.

Johns, H. (1996) *Personal development in counsellor training*. London: Cassell.

Lennie, C. (2007) "The role of personal development groups in counsellor training: Understanding factors contributing to self-awareness in the personal development group." *British Journal of Guidance & Counselling* 35(1): 115–129.

Levine, S. K. (1988) *Foundations of expressive arts therapy: Theoretical and clinical perspectives*. London: Jessica Kingsley.

Levine, S. K. (1992) *Poiesis: The language of psychology and the speech of the soul*. London: Jessica Kingsley.

Madison, S. D. (2012) *Critical ethnography: Method, ethics, and performance studies*. Los Angeles: Sage Publications.

McKenzie-Mavinga, I. (2005) *A study of black issues in counsellor training* 2002–2005. DProf thesis, Middlesex University, London.

McNeilly, G. (2006) *Group Analytic Art Therapy*. London; Jessica Kingsley.

McNiff, S. (1998) *Trust the process: An artist's guide to letting go*. Boston: Shambhala Publication Inc.

McWilliams, N. (2004) *Psychoanalytic psychotherapy: A practitioner's guide*. New York: Guilford Press.

Moore, K., and K. Marder. (2020) *Mentalizing in group art therapy: Interventions for emerging adults*. London: Jessica Kingsley.

Rose, C. (2008) *The personal development group: The students guide*. London: Karnac Books.

Tatum, B. D. (1997). *Why are all the Black kids sitting together in the cafeteria?* New York: Basic Books.

Talwar, S. (2019) *Art therapy for social justice, radical intersections*. Abingdon: Routledge.

Waller, D. (2015) *Group interactive art therapy: Its use in training and treatment*. Abingdon: Routledge.

Winnicott, D. W. (1971) *Playing and reality*. Harmondsworth: Penguin.

Chapter 11

Untold stories – the art of imagination in later life

Storytelling and multi-modal arts psychotherapy on an older adult inpatient mental health ward

Rebecca Smart and Jack Eastwood

> We walk up the corridor slowly. This is unknown territory. Feet shuffle, a walking frame taps the floor, the clang of doors, a distant alarm. A pause at the door, a clatter of keys, a turn in the lock. We go in. There is music playing. A table with a bright silk scarf in the middle with objects on it. Paints, pastels, pens, paper. Colour. And the trees, let's not forget the trees. A room flooded with light and trees all around.
>
> (Memory vignette)

This is a story of how a group came together, once a week, to share stories in this room. Stories from the old days, stories from around the world, stories from long remembered lives. How those stories were listened to, talked about, and then translated into art – drawings, paintings, images. How the art was seen, responded to, and made into a poem. Words that held some of the shapes of the untold stories that ran like an undercurrent through that room.

The story that we will tell in this chapter is set in an older adult functional ward within a large inner city mental health hospital. It is an exploration of an open multi-modal storytelling and arts psychotherapies group ran once a week over a period of four years, with Rebecca Smart, an integrative arts psychotherapist, and Jack Eastwood, a Drama Psychotherapist. The work was devised collaboratively, in a multi-layered integrative approach – integration of creative practices within a dual modality partnership, integration of different art forms, and integration of theories including Attachment theory (Bowlby, Holmes, Wallin), Winnicott, Clarkson's Five Relationships, Gestalt, Jung, and current trauma informed practice and neuroscience (Siegal, Van der Kolk, Herman).

There are layers to this story, nested inside each other like Russian dolls. Our multi-modal arts psychotherapy group sat within the context of the medical model. Complex trauma ran beneath the many medical diagnoses we worked with, which included psychosis, bi-polar, anxiety disorders, clinical depression, schizo-affective disorder, personality disorders. Trauma informed practice was central, with a focus on empowerment, choice, community and collaboration.

DOI: 10.4324/9781003155676-16

As Van Der Kolk (2014) points out: *"Being a patient, rather than a participant in one's healing process, separates suffering people from their community and alienates them from an inner sense of self"* (p. 38). Balancing the need for regulation of affect whilst also offering a space where untold stories could find expression without causing re-traumatisation, underpinned our way of working.

We will be inviting you into a "storying" of the group experience, to offer a felt sense of how different creative processes wove together to create an artistic space where the group could connect. Fragments of poetry from the words of group members will be included throughout, so that their voices can be heard from the heart of the work.

Rites of Passage and Later Life

One of the group poems captures something of the experience of the invisibility of old age, drawing on nature as a metaphor:

> *The changing of the trees and the leaves*
> *The beginning of the change*
> *It doesn't all happen at once*
> *It happens over a time*
> *You can't draw wind.*
>
> (Group Poem 1)

Part of the task of this group was to allow the invisible to become visible, in a way that could be bearable. The existential pain of this time of life, facing what Yalom (1980) identifies as the four "givens" of existence – death, isolation, meaning in life, and freedom – demanded a genuine meeting.

> Yalom (2001) writes that "our life, our existence, will always be riveted to death, love to loss, freedom to fear, and growth to separation. We are, all of us, in this together"
>
> (p. 14).

The group poetry elicited by the art images became a place where people's experience of losses could be shared:

> *Tree of life*
>
> *You can put a heart on it*
> *To remember someone*
>
> *You loved and lost.*
>
> *My strength is weak*

I can't walk any more
I'd love to be able to walk
I want to be able to live life to the full

We tried that's all we can say

We tried.

(Group Poem 2)

For older adults entering the mental health ward, there has been a shedding of identity on multiple levels, a bereavement of selves. Possible losses include loss of role within a job, loss of loved ones and family, loss of position within a community, physical and cognitive abilities, and a subsequent toll of loneliness and isolation. To frame this in the context of a rite of passage, Turner (1965: 95) describes liminal space as being "betwixt and between", where the person "passes through a realm that has few or none of the attributes of the past or coming state". In this space between past and future, the liminal is a space where previous identity has been shed, where 'the state of the ritual subject . . . is ambiguous' (Turner, 1965: 94). Stepping into the liminal is to walk into a time of transition, a state of disorientation where nothing is as it once was, and what will be is unknown.

Contextualising the inpatient stay as being a 'liminal' experience within a wider rite of passage acknowledges that there has been a separation, a severance from a previous way of life. Van Gennep (in Turner, 1965: 94) identifies 3 stages – separation, limen, and incorporation. The ward itself can be framed as a liminal space where people exist in a halfway place between admission (separation) and discharge (return/incorporation). The liminal nature of being both at a transitional stage of life in older age, whilst also being placed within the 'betwixt and between' (Turner, 1965: 95) world of the mental health ward, can sharpen the experience of being cast outside 'ordinary life'.

The medical experience involves ward routines, medication, new structures and unfamiliar staff, institutionalised spaces and unfamiliar companions. This can all contribute to a sense of being unmoored from anchors that offer a sense of self in the wider world. A metaphor that arose when thinking of the ward, was of people cast adrift at sea in need of a haven – a place to drop anchor, to land. Part of the function of the group was to provide a place where members could also reflect on their ward experience, which in itself could be experienced as a traumatic dislocation. Our intention was to offer a therapeutic space that felt invitational, creative, welcoming. The structure of the group would become like a rite of passage in itself – separating from the ward, taking the journey into the liminal space of the arts therapies room, then returning back to the ward having shared a creative experience together.

Arts as an Anchor

One key goal of the group was to offer a place where people could anchor their sense of innate "personhood" within this liminal experience. Kitwood (1997) describes personhood as: ". . . *a standing or status that is bestowed upon one human being, by others, in the context of relationship and social being. It implies recognition, respect and trust*" (p. 8). The possible erosion of a sense of personhood within the limbo of an institutional setting can be actively countered through a trauma-informed arts psychotherapies approach:

1   **Creativity:** The loss of a sense of personal value in the world can be met by the possibility of creativity – creating something from nothing, which is then treated as something to be respected and valued.
2   **Choice**: Loss of autonomy can be worked within the many decision-making moments during art making, where someone is offered the opportunity and support to regain personal authority in making active choices.
3   **Community**: Loss of a sense of community – a sense of being adrift amidst strangers, can be met by the connection of a group sharing an artistic focus, a common creative endeavour.
4   **Communication**: The ability to communicate, to express an inner world to others, can be met by different modes of expression, where story, art, and poetry can point to experiences that may be too difficult to meet head-on.

Creative collaboration – myth and nature

Working as co-therapists offered a rich opportunity to integrate dual modality working, with our different backgrounds as drama psychotherapist and integrative arts psychotherapist. At the time, Jack was in his 60s, Rebecca was in her 40s. We were both white British, middle class, living in a rural area. This similarity of background contrasted with the diversity within the groups we ran. Thinking about how our positions within the group could be seen in the context of power and privilege, and enabling voices that could experience marginalisation to be heard, was an ongoing part of the work. There were some core creative commonalities between us – we both came from theatre backgrounds and have a love of improvisation and play. The key that unlocked our way of working together was our shared love of storytelling.

Both of us are storytellers who, in our own personal creative process, have explored the embodied relationship between image, symbol, and myth through working with stories in the woods. Relating to the "more than human world" can be an invitation to slow down to hear a deeper kind of language, to open up the imaginal world, and to experience wider synchronicity. The Forest brings layers of encounter, which can reflect and amplify the dance between the unconscious and the mythic. Mary-Jayne Rust (in Siddons Heginworth & Nash, 2020) writes:

> The forest offers many teachings: the art of being deeply rooted in place, or the art of shedding skin. . . . This is a place where the soul can be spoken to and recharged, where the rational mind can let go and allow a more playful spirit in.
>
> (p. xvi)

We wondered how our personal creative approaches to storytelling, inviting relationship with nature, play, and imagination, could inform the clinical practice on the ward?

There were a few key principles that fed into the ward work. First, the idea of stories calling people back to themselves, restoring a sense of identity and community through a shared listening experience. Second, the importance of the wider field of the "more than human world" – the seasons, the trees, and the sense of place that surrounds the storytelling. And third, the imagery from the story having some space to be expressed and reflected on through encounter, to allow the unconscious, the unspoken, to find a different language. In this instance, this would be through layers of different art forms and sharing stories within the group.

The therapeutic space

Paying attention to the natural world within the institutional environment was made possible by the multi-purpose therapy room, which was away from the ward. Surrounded by windows, one side looked over the garden, the other into the woods bordering a nature reserve. The trees, the changing seasons, the squirrels, and the birds were all part of the experience.

> We walk through the door into music, art on table, trees all around. Like a hut in the middle of the woods. It has been a long walk to get here, but we made it. We sit around a table and settle. There is a lot to take in. Paints and pebbles from the beach, the sound of music from the past, the freshly sprung blossoms on the cherry tree by the window. Water is poured into cups, and we arrive.
>
> (Memory vignette)

Setting out on the journey

The journey to the room involved stepping over the threshold of the ward, taking a walk to a completely different space. For some group members, this leap took courage. Once in the therapy room, the creative experience also involved taking risks, each engagement with art forms another step into the unknown. Risk assessment took place before the group began, consulting with the wider ward team, and engaging with individuals on the ward. It was an open trans-diagnostic group, and risk assessment was ongoing and dynamic within the sessions. Siegel's (1999) concept of working within the "window of tolerance", noticing hypo and hyper arousal and trauma reactions, supported us to continually assess the level of affect that was being experienced so that we could grade the arts to establish a sense of containment and holding.

Each session had a clear structure within which the different art forms wove, like a dance of call and response, each act of creativity a reflection and amplification of the last. Whilst the structure was defined, each part of the session could be expanded or curtailed depending on the needs of the participants. Yalom (2001) writes: "therapy is spontaneous, the relationship is dynamic and ever-evolving, and there is a continuous sequence of experiencing and then examining the process. At its very core, the flow of therapy should be spontaneous, forever following unanticipated riverbeds" (p. 34).

Somatic observation of the group throughout every stage of the arts process and having flexibility to change and grade as we went along was key to the work. We watched out for overwhelm or dissociation, using grounding and re-orientating to the room in the "here and now" to build security. The sense of pride that group members gradually developed in managing the journey to the room, and in their creative process, reflected an expansion of their "window of tolerance" (Siegel, 1999) through daring to step into the many unknowns this experience offered and finding it to be safe enough.

1. Arrival

The initial phase of the session was Arrival. The focus was on bridging the group members into the room and introducing a creative space. Welcoming, grounding, and playing host to the imagination were part of this. Music was played, and this was talked about, sometimes altered for different tastes. Water was poured and given out. We would draw attention to the environment, the trees, the garden, and the sounds of the room. Something from nature in the centre of the table often acted as a source of inspiration for art making:

> *This is the spindle tree*
> *Gorgeous*
> *Like fireworks*
> *It fills the page*
> *It's got presence*
>   (Group poem 3)

Objects related to the story were also placed in the centre. We chose objects that inspired curiosity, inviting the group to focus on "what is this?" A shark's tooth, a giant bobbin from a loom, an unusual feather – passed around from hand to hand with suggestions. Play and curiosity, together with sensory experience of touching and examining, helped to ground and to encourage a mindful awareness of the present moment. We also used this to assess levels of anxiety/arousal within the group.

2. Storytelling

The next stage was Storytelling. We would often start with a simple folk tale that had themes that would help to connect and stabilise the group. If the group was robust enough, we could introduce stories that held more challenge and depth.

An ongoing theme in this open group was beginnings and endings, with discharge and the transience of home a central concern for people. One story we often told around times of ending was centred around the sea. The "warm-up" exercise was to hold and mindfully explore pebbles from the beach, which became a sensory anchor to ground throughout the session. After checking in and listening to the personal stories evoked by the warm-up, we would ask if they were ready to listen to a story.

"The Woman and the Star" is about a woman who leaves the safety of her home where she lives alone, to follow the sound of a singing star:

> Such a song. It calls to her, pulling her from a walk to a run, past the home she loves, through the forest she loves, to the beach. She steps into her boat and pushes away from the shore. Then she looks back, back at this land that she knows so well. How do you leave the land you love? The star sings. Hooks around her heart. She puts her paddle in the water, and she rows, and she rows . . . always following that star.
>
> (Excerpt adapted from an Aboriginal tale,
> originally heard in a telling by
> Sophia Condaris, drama therapist)

This story held multiple layers. The themes of leaving and arrival offered the group an opportunity to explore their own current experience of hospital admission and future discharge, within the safety of the metaphor of the woman's story. It also spoke to the courage needed to step over thresholds into new places – which they had all just done in stepping off the ward and into the therapy room. We offered a reflective space to see where they were pulled to in the story, what they thought of the woman's journey, and what she might be feeling. We then shifted into a non-verbal exploration of the story through art and imagery.

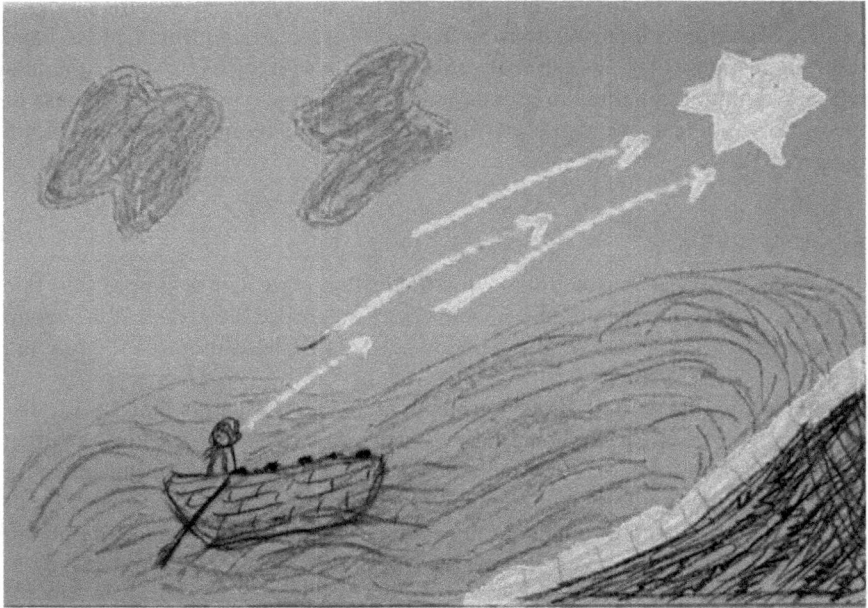

Figure 11.1 Following the star. Oil pastel on paper

3. Art

The third stage was Art making. One of the choices offered was an invitation to paint, draw or collage an image from the story.

One group member drew a boat with arrows pointing towards the star to represent the sense of determination she noticed in the story:

> *She's following the star in the boat*
> *She's got it in her*
> *To do what she feels she should*
> *By following the star*
> (Group Poem 4)

Another group member disclosed that her husband had died when she was a young mother, and that she had no time to grieve. For her, painting the star in the story reminded her of telling her child that Dad had become a star in the sky:

At the end of the art making, she reflected on her image with the group, and some of her words were captured in the group poem:

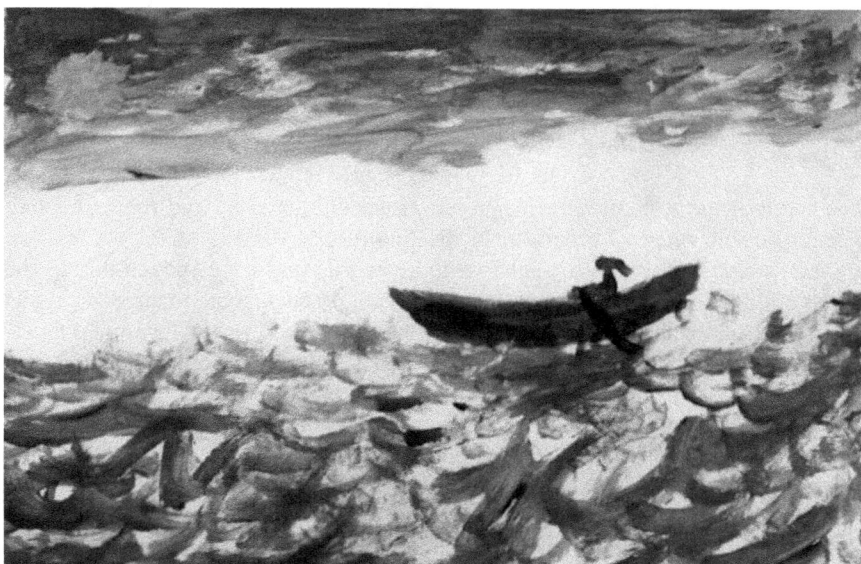

Figure 11.2 A better place. Acrylic on paper

She's going to a better place
Following the star
Somewhere that might be better
We don't know what's round the corner
Do we?
Sense of hope and bravery
(Group Poem 5)

The vulnerability of the lone woman rowing in the image contrasts with the hope of the words in the poem, whilst the phrase "better place" holds connotations of death. A transpersonal aspect of the work was how the often-unspoken subject of death wove through the different art forms. It was present and visible in the shifting seasons of nature around us, and the stories, art, and poetry offered opportunities to hold, often unconsciously, the many bereavements and the experience of the approaching end of life within the group.

Art making was graded to allow for the wide diversity in reactions that the invitation to paint or draw evoked. Collage was a way in for those too intimidated by the idea of painting, and those who did not want to make could choose to carry on discussing the stories instead. Making an image of a calm place, or object that connected to a sense of being "OK enough" was a way of grounding and stabilising at the start of the work. Sharing images with each other at the end and having time to reflect on what the images evoked offered an opportunity for creativity to be witnessed in a non-judgemental and supportive way.

4. Poetry

The fourth stage was included when the group felt cohesive and robust enough to engage with one last art form. In the final group sharing of the art images, we would ask permission to speed write keywords that were spoken during the group's reflections. This formed an improvised, spontaneous poem, which was then read back to the group. Each section was verbally directed towards the person whose image had elicited the words. The room became silent, everyone paying attention, often with moments of nodding and recognition. It is hard to express the quality of shared attention at this moment. Helene Cixous (1998, as cited by Tufnell and Crickmay, 2004: 63), captures something of this quality, when she writes: "I do not write to keep. I write to feel. I write to touch the body of the instant with the tips of words".

The power of the poem was in the meeting between the act of speaking, and the feeling that was generated in the group in the act of listening – what Buber (1970) would describe as an "I-Thou" moment. It evoked a stillness, a shared attention, and a sense that we had all created something together:

> *We are all artists and don't know it*
> *Clouds in squares of sky*
> (Group Poem 6)

The process of scribing only words spoken by the group members, with nothing else added, offered the group ownership of the spoken words. The poem was a mirroring of the many layers of imaginative participation within the session and served as a satisfying full stop to the creative process, an offering of soul food. This transpersonal dimension was a core aspect of the arts psychotherapies journey. Rollo May (1975) writes that this type of experience gives: "a sharpened perception, a vividness, a translucence of relationship to the things around us. The world becomes vivid and unforgettable" (p. 61).

The combination of the art image and the poem enabled group members to have a sense of being both seen and heard, their hidden stories held in paint and poetry:

> *Sunrise or sunset?*
> *Which way?*
> *The rays of the sun*
> *The golden coin that fell in the river*
> *It's quite hidden*
> *But it can be seen.*
> (Group Poem 7)

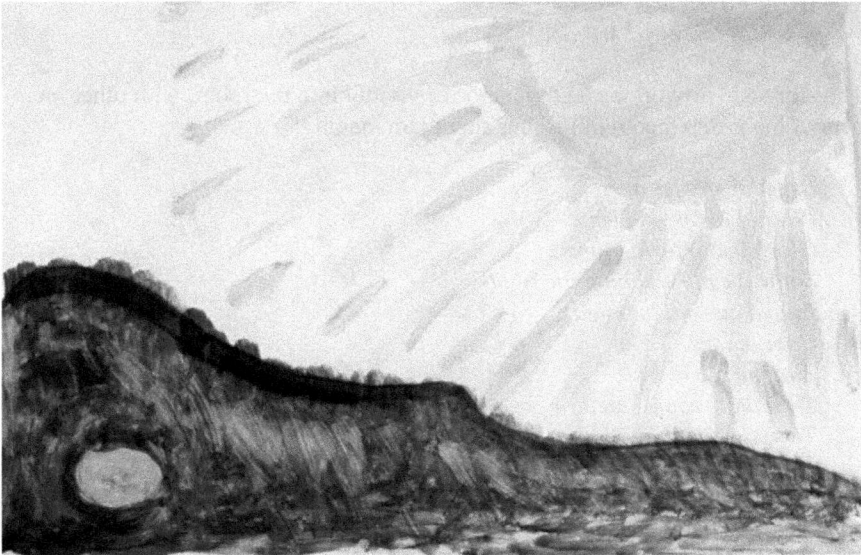

Figure 11.3 Hidden but seen. Acrylic on paper

Later, with the group's permission, we would go back to the ward and give members a copy of the poem – perhaps acting as a transitional object (Winnicott, 1951) to connect back to the creativity and holding of the group.

Connection through reminiscence

The various art forms were a way of supporting clients to anchor back to times and places they found resourceful, as well as an opportunity to express and share feelings that could not be verbalised. One session we chose to tell a Russian Gypsy Tale (Riordan 2002: 73) which held a theme of finding the sweetness in bitter experiences, through the metaphor of berries and fruit. Traditional stories can speak to diverse people from different backgrounds and find points of connection that are unexpected. One group member reminisced about his childhood as a traveller:

> *To survive*
> *We'd go place to place*
> *Hop picking apple picking*
> *Plums*
> *You name it we did it*
> *Very free*

We just loved it
We just lived it
(Group Poem 8)

The story and artwork brought memories vividly into the room, with other members of the group then reminiscing about jam making:

Bramley apples
Piles of black berries
Glorious Victoria plums
Shiny purple catching the light
Boiled cooked bubbled
Cool in jars
A big urn
The whole room smelling
Then the tasting bit
The best bit
Nice and clean
The fruit that's ready
Lovely flow
Sweetness and bitterness
Biting into the bitter fruit
Nature is constantly beautiful.
(Group Poem 9)

In this session, the story, art making, and the poem all interwove to create a vivid experience of connection with past stories that linked to memories of freedom in nature, childhood play, and sensory pleasure. Holmes (1993) points out the importance of therapy in providing the security for narrative competence to emerge: "It creates out of fragmentary experience an unbroken line or thread. . . . Narrative gives a person a sense of ownership of their past and their life" (p. 150). The poem reflects the paradoxical experience of "sweetness and bitterness" existing side by side within the session itself – these past narratives being shared within a mental health hospital when group members were indeed "biting into the bitter fruit". The use of metaphor enabled pain to be referred to obliquely, a sideways glance, a subtle acknowledgment of the difficulty underlying the sweetness that had been explored in the reminiscing.

Art making and shame

Attachment theory informed our thinking around the creative process – Holmes (1993) states that a key quality of a secure relationship is active, reciprocal interaction. Our aim was to introduce the arts in a way that encouraged a sense of agency, autonomy, and ability to make decisions, particularly necessary for this age group. This involved encouraging play, which as Winnicott (1971) pointed out, should be spontaneous rather than compliant: "where playing is not possible then the work done by the therapist is directed toward bringing the patient from a state of not being able to play into a state of being able to play" (p. 68). Play involves risk – the unknown, getting it "wrong", a fear of failure, the possibility of shame.

The need to establish safety, to meet clients with empathic attunement, and offer permission giving both in terms of the art making and in the expression of feelings during the sessions, was key to working with shame. The tension between fear of failure and the acceptance offered by this approach to the art making was expressed in one of the group poems:

The stages of drawing
Pencilling it in, firming it up
After the tentative lines
Overcoming perfectionism
When something's not quite right
Then you accept it as not quite right
And enjoy it.
It's good enough.
                    (Group Poem 10)

However, for some, "good enough" might not be an accessible feeling. One group member had a recent diagnosis of a terminal disease, which impacted his ability to make art as he had once been able to. He had drawn a faint pencil image of Hokusai's *Great Wave* that could barely be seen. Reflecting on his image, the words he spoke were captured in the group poem:

It reminds me how life can be so harsh
How much I'm missing now
The joy of the world
There was a time when I would be
Fascinated
Join in.
A sadness
That I can't join in.
I was a wordsmith once
It's frustrating
Tiny little things are too much.
                    (Group Poem 11)

In terms of Clarkson's therapeutic relationship model (1995), the Reparative Relationship was of central importance. Lapworth and Sills (2010) write that meta-analysis of psychotherapy outcome research identifying common factors of successful therapy are largely related to: "the existence, from the client's point of view, of an empathic, respectful relationship that remains accepting and non-judgmental, even after the client has exposed the parts of herself that she experiences as flawed or shameful" (p. 18). Our task as therapists was to provide "good enough" (Winnicott, 1953) therapeutic holding, so that difficult emotions that might emerge during the creative process could find a space to be expressed and acknowledged.

Integration of Multiple Art Forms

The integration of multiple art forms enabled clients' experiences to find varying forms of expression within creative medium. The reading of the poem at the end of a session was the culmination of a series of creative responses which fed back to the group their own words, their own experiences. Bion (1967) describes a mother receiving an infant's fears and responding, "in a manner that makes the infant feel it is receiving its frightened personality back again but in a form that it can tolerate" (p. 104). There was a dance of call and response between the art forms that offered layers of mirroring, validation, and affect attunement.

The interweaving of music, sensory objects, storytelling, art making, and poetry placed a focus on creativity throughout the sessions, which supported a sense of shared attention and community. Each engagement was graded to offer grounding and resource, and to support a sense of autonomy and active choice making. The multi-layered creative processes enabled us to hold the tension between the sense of safety needed for trauma informed treatment, whilst also offering the opportunity for the untold stories within the group to emerge through encounter with the arts.

Endings

Marion Woodman (in Mahdi, Foster & Little, 1987) writes of the need to accept

> the slow, unhurried, cyclic rhythms of nature, which allow time for birth, maturation, and death. When some part of us dies, there must be a time of mourning, a period of withdrawal and introspection, a period of allowing the tears to fall.
>
> (p. 211)

Contextualising the inpatient work with older adults as a rite of passage frames the therapeutic encounter as existing in a time where the individual exists "betwixt and between" different worlds of experience. The therapy room becomes a liminal space, which can hold the dissolution and disintegration of what has gone before, whilst creativity itself points to the possibility that something new can emerge. The many stories that were held in the shapes of paint, poetry, and image, acted as a bridge between the unconscious and the expression of emotion, allowing some of what felt unbearable to be born, acknowledged, and met within the arts psychotherapies group.

References

Bion, W.R. (1967). *Second Thoughts*. London: William Heinemann Medical Books Ltd.

Buber, M. (1970). *I and Thou*. New York: Touchstone.

Clarkson, P. (1995). *The Therapeutic Relationship*. London: Whurr Publishers Ltd.

Holmes, J. (1993). *John Bowlby and Attachment Theory*. London: Routledge.

Kitwood, T. (1997). *Dementia Reconsidered: The Person Comes First*. Buckingham: Open University Press.

Lapworth, P. and Sills, C. (2010). *Integration in Counselling and Psychotherapy, 2nd Edition: Developing a Personal Approach*. London: Sage Publications Ltd.

Mahdi, L.C., Foster, S. and Little, M. (1987). *Betwixt and Between: Patterns of Masculine and Feminine Initiation*. La Salle, IL: Open Court.

May, R. (1975). *The Courage to Create*. New York: Norton.

Riordan, J. (2002). *Russian Gypsy Tales*. New York: Interlink Publishing Group.

Siddons Heginworth, I. and Nash, G. (2020). *Environmental Arts Therapy: The Wild Frontiers of the Heart*. Abingdon: Routledge.

Siegel, D.J. (1999). *The Developing Mind: Toward a Neurobiology of Interpersonal Experience*. New York: Guilford Press.

Tufnell, M. and Crickmay, C. (2004). *A Widening Field: Journeys in Body and Imagination*. Hampshire: Dance Books.

Turner, V. (1965). *The Ritual Process: Structure and Anti-Structure*. Ithaca: Cornell University Press.

Van Der Kolk, B. (2014). *The Body Keeps the Score*. New York: Viking Penguin.

Winnicott, D.W. (1951). *Transitional Objects and Transitional Phenomena. Collected Papers: Through Paediatrics to Psycho-analysis*. London: Tavistock Publication.

Winnicott, D.W. (1953). Transitional Objects and Transitional Phenomena – A Study of the First Not-Me Possession. *International Journal of Pscyho-Analysis*, vol. 34, pp. 89–97.

Winnicott, D.W. (1971). *Playing and Reality*. Abingdon: Routledge.

Yalom, I.D. (1980). *Existential Psychotherapy*. New York: Basic Books.

Yalom, I.D. (2001). *The Gift of Therapy*. London: Piatkus Books.

Chapter 12

Creating an integrative arts psychotherapy group treatment model to support people with a dual diagnosis in residential rehab

RAFT (Recovery and Aftercare from Formative Trauma)

Sarah Hall

Introduction and Context

The metaphor "all at sea" is a ubiquitous mien at Chy rehab, where patients typically arrive from detox, feeling completely lost or deeply confused. Located in Cornwall, Chy is surrounded by sea, but the etymology of this nautical idiom heralds from a time before modern navigational systems, when a ship was out of sight of land, in a dangerous, uncertain position. Correspondingly, a "night sea journey" is an archetypal motif in mythology, psychologically associated with depression and the loss of energy, characteristic of neurosis (Jung, 1936). Mythologically, the night sea journey motif usually involves being swallowed by a dragon or sea monster, but could equally translate to being consumed by addiction.

Rehab is considered a lifeline by those seeking to salvage their lives from the ravages of addiction, a final attempt to reach the shore after a perilous voyage alone at sea. The collective experience gained by working as an integrative arts psychotherapist in residential rehabs, as well as personal recovery from addiction, led me to develop an integrative arts psychotherapy programme known as RAFT (*Recovery and Aftercare from Formative Trauma*). This programme provides specific support for people with a dual diagnosis and/or trauma history, who face additional challenges in overcoming addiction, particularly during the tempestuous stages of early recovery. The structure, content, and integrative arts modality were informed by feedback from multiple service users, who having reached the safe haven of rehab, continued to struggle to stay afloat.

Chy is a secondary care residential rehab, operated by *'We Are With You'*, (formerly Addaction), a charity with over 40 years' experience in providing drug, alcohol, and mental health services throughout England and Scotland. The rehab has 18 residential beds providing 24/7 care, with treatment typically lasting between 3 and 6 months. Chy accepts multi-cultural and mixed gender referrals

DOI: 10.4324/9781003155676-17

from across the UK, with residents drawn from community drug and alcohol services, the criminal justice system, the homeless community, mental health services, and the private sector.

Therapeutic Community

Chy was founded on the principles of a Therapeutic Community, which is distinct from a 12-step fellowship, or mutual aid approach to addiction and recovery. The concept of Therapeutic Community has a diverse history including communities that teach, heal, and support; in religious sects and utopian communes, and in spiritual, temperance, and mental health reform movements (De Leon, 2000: 12), with early models of communal healing and support dating back to classical antiquity. The current treatment model at Chy blends a classic therapeutic community approach, with contemporary psychotherapy modalities, psycho-education, and psychiatry.

Design considerations

The rationale for creating an integrative arts psychotherapy model stemmed from the need to address participants' different psychological injuries, and cultural influences, within a time-limited group therapy format. Harnessing an integrative approach (Clarkson, 2003), with a unifying multi-dimensional relational framework, enabled the development of interventions and healing across all six relationship modes (Gilbert and Orlans, 2010). The central role of the arts in expounding unconscious communications additionally amplified both the personal and collective understanding of complexes (Jung, 1969), which had hitherto been hidden, or too traumatic to speak of.

I considered multifarious definitions of addiction with which different individuals identified, ensuring relevance and buy-in, including: physiological dependence, tolerance, and withdrawal; behaviour that is centrifugal; substance use or behaviour that persists despite negative consequences; life that becomes unmanageable; addictive behaviours which assume control of the person; and distorted thinking/behaving leading to irrational thoughts, unmanageable feelings, and self-defeating behaviours. Khantzian's (2012: 274–279) view that "addiction is not about pleasure seeking; nor is it about human self-destructiveness or oral dependency – as some well-accepted formulations suggest, but rather an attempt at self-correction that fails", underpinning them all.

Due to the prevalence of dual diagnosis patients accessing rehab, mental health conditions/symptoms, including complex-trauma, post-traumatic-stress-disorder, drug-induced/organic psychosis, depression, anxiety, and personality disorders, necessitated specific consideration of both intrapsychic and interpersonal aspects of psychological functioning. The therapeutic metier of the programme consequently evolved to address unconscious defences, body dysmorphic disorder, repetition compulsion, cravings and triggers, flashbacks, panic attacks/anxiety, nightmares and intrusive thoughts, dysregulation/mood instability and self-harm, anger, grief, loss and isolation, dissociation/derealisation, shame and guilt, psychosomatic illnesses, denial, and depression.

Although this programme development preceded my training as a Jungian Analyst, reading about Jung's clinical work with addiction emphasised the primacy of the transpersonal therapeutic process. Having described alcoholism as "a spiritual thirst for wholeness", Jung (1961) posited that "only a radical conversion to something equally satisfying to the individual at a deep level could promote lasting recovery". Suggesting that psychological development extends to include higher states of consciousness and can continue throughout life, Jung proposed that transcendent experience lies within, is accessible to everyone, and that the healing and growth stimulated by such experience often make use of the languages of symbolic imagery and nonverbal experience. As Clarkson (2003) has also explained, the transpersonal relationship can be seen to permeate the work of creativity, healing, growth, and dying, giving credence to its core inclusion.

The shapeshifting capacity of integrative arts psychotherapy

The validity of art therapy as an effective treatment for addiction has been widely established (Moore, 1983); however, an explicit integrative arts psychotherapy approach for dual diagnosis has not. Art therapy treatment for addiction has largely been evaluated on its efficacy with single theoretical paradigms, such as psychodynamic therapy (Albert-Puleo, 1980) or 12-step treatment models, (Julliard, 1995). Other studies have focused on particular groups, or problems in addictions treatment, such as gender (Hanes, 2017); families (Callaghan, 1993); themes like ambivalence (Horay, 2006) and narcissism (Lachman-Chapin, 1979); shame (Johnson, 1990); and resistance (Springham, 1998).

With the ambitious remit of RAFT, resembling the contents of Pandora's jar/box, it became clear a multi-faceted cache of therapeutic responses was required. The multiple theoretical frameworks and integrated application of all the arts, involved in an integrative arts psychotherapy approach, emerged as optimal, due in part to its integral shapeshifting potential. In mythology/folklore, shapeshifting is the ability to physically transform, be it through an inherently superhuman ability, divine intervention, demonic manipulation, or the use of sorcery/spells; the idea of shapeshifting is the oldest form of shamanism. Thus, an integrative arts psychotherapy model capable of holding the layers of therapy in mind, and using these to unite multiple theories with manifold art forms and interventions, offered the requisite flexibility.

The prescribed group therapy format additionally benefited from the shapeshifting capacity of this approach. Group treatment modalities are almost universally the preferred or predominant therapeutic modality for patients with substance use disorders (Flores, 2007; Matano and Yalom, 1991). The justification, often erroneously attributed to financial constraints or motives, in fact stems from the group's augmented ability to counteract isolation, its prowess in facilitating interpersonal opportunities for healing shame and rehearsing new ways of being; dual qualities that promote the culture of recovery (Herman, 1992; Yalom, 1985). Consequently, the RAFT programmes' ability to blend wide-ranging theoretical and practice-based methods, with the dynamic curative factors of group therapy which include: altruism, catharsis, cohesiveness, confrontation, existentiality, family re-enactment, hope, identification, insight, and universality, render it uniquely placed to influence the complex causes and symptoms of addiction.

The integrative arts shapeshifting nature of the programme also offered a solution to the plural demographic challenges, overcoming variances in participants' psychological readiness by simultaneously operating at different depths and levels of understanding, emulating the various stages of alchemy, linked by Jung to the psychological process of "Individuation". Jung explains:

> Only after I had familiarised myself with alchemy did I realise that the unconscious is a **process**, and that the psyche is transformed or developed by the relationship of the ego to the contents of the unconscious.
>
> (Schwartz-Salant, 1995: 235)

Individuation, in Jungian psychology, is the process whereby an individual realises a state of spiritual and psychological wholeness. Through this process, that, which was previously fragmented and broken, is restored and synthesised so that a whole and unique individual emerges.

> The process by which a person becomes a psychological "in-dividual", that is a separate, indivisible unity or "whole".
>
> (Jung, 1934/1954/1981, CW Vol. 9, p. 275)

Alchemy and integrative arts psychotherapy

In "Jungian Arts-Based Research" (Rowland and Weishaus, 2021), Rowland identifies the processes of alchemy as a valuable research methodology. Art therapy shares many affiliations with alchemy. On an external level, both disciplines interact with materials to generate a final product, while on an internal level, both seek to promote insight and change within the individuals engaged in their processes. Integrative arts psychotherapy has an additional affinity with alchemy in that it combines different creative art forms/materials and theoretical modalities to assist the psyche in the service of transformation, analogous to Alchemy's use of metals/substances, rituals, and imagination in pursuit of the philosopher's gold or stone. This alchemical transformation of matter and mind has been expressed through the four stages of *Nigredo* (black), *Albedo* (white), *Citrinitas* (yellow), and *Rubedo* (red), collectively comprising the processes of *calcination, solutio, separatio, coniunctio, putrefaction, coagulatio, cibatio, sublimation, fermentation, exaltation, augmentatio*, and *projection* (Jung, 1944).

In art therapy language, McNiff (1988) maintains that the art materials themselves provide the art therapy process with a structure and that their specific natures influence the outcome, with substrate, scale, medium, tools, and even the smell of art supplies all being essential elements. Correspondingly, Moon (1997) maintains that making visible objects out of inner images in art therapy provides an opportunity to achieve balance between our inner and outer experiences. Coining the term "meta-verbal" modality of intervention, Moon (1994), describes how the four interactions between the client-artist, the media, the procedure, and the art therapist, combine to create a modality which is beyond words and teaches by living through processes, rather than by talking. This is a view endorsed by Jung (2009/1875–1961: 123): "I speak in images. With nothing else can I express the words from the depths".

In the RAFT programme, the influence of alchemy not only applies to the specific multimedia interventions but also extends to the ordering process of the 16 sessions, reflecting the procedural metaphor of turning lead (dual diagnosis symptoms) into gold (psychological individuation).

RAFT as a semi-structured model

Detailed consideration of the evidence base relating to addiction, dual diagnosis, and trauma, was augmented with clinical experience of art therapy in residential rehab settings and private practice, as well as personal lived experience of addiction and recovery. The result was a 16-session, twice-weekly, semi-structured programme.

Concern has been voiced about art therapy which endorses a "*directional, prescriptive approach*", in contrast to a non-directive, psychodynamic, patient-led tradition of art therapy (Mahony and Waller, 1992). However, given the characteristically chaotic internal world and disordered behaviours associated with early recovery and dual diagnosis, the bespoke semi-structured arts-based interventions used in RAFT act as a navigational guide, facilitating engagement with affect recognition/regulation, self-esteem, interpersonal dynamics, and self-care problems in a graded and containing way. The shapeshifting properties of the integrative approach additionally permit participants to respond intuitively to the session-by-session leitmotifs, engendering meaningful authentic individual retorts, within the overall programme framework. The semi-structured format also supports the co-facilitation, given that the discomforting and disorganising aspects of addiction, trauma, and dual diagnosis can disrupt both those experiencing the symptoms, as well as those who vicariously witness them. The therapeutic community also supports the clinical delivery by serving as an additional attachment figure (Flores, 2001).

RAFT is a closed group, averaging 12–15 participants, facilitated by an art therapist and co-facilitator. Attendance is not compulsory, but all residents are encouraged to participate. The residential context is pertinent given the expectation of delivering meaningful change for participants with dual diagnosis in just

8 weeks, necessitating a depth psychology approach to short-term therapy, which an integrative arts approach delivers.

The RAFT clinical sessions

Week 1: "Active Imagination" (Calcinatio)

The initial focus is on establishing the creative foundations of RAFT, using Active Imagination, a Jungian technique for bridging conscious and unconscious expression by giving free reign to fantasy, while simultaneously maintaining an active, attentive, conscious point of view (Chodorow, 1997). Selecting from 200 archetypal postcard images covering the floor, participants use a combination of focus, meditation, and imaginative association, to animate the symbols/images, allowing unconscious expression. A personal image based on the experience is then created, and after returning to normal conscious awareness, the image is discussed with the group. The process creates an embodied synthesis of conscious/unconscious material captured in an image and is retained as a grounding tool should anyone become dissociated or dysregulated during the subsequent sessions; the image acts as a safe anchor or transitional object (Winnicott, 1953).

In the second session, the emphasis is on sharing personal narratives through the collaborative production and playing of a giant board game. This intervention solicits information on historical coping strategies and encourages exploration of collective script patterns and inter-generational schemas that may be dominating the psyche. The game uses animal symbolism to enhance the flow of unconscious projections and feelings (Case, 2005), while also pushing participants to risk imagining their futures.

Week 2: "Establishing Foundations for Change" (Separatio)

This session highlights repetition compulsion/fixed gestalts, which commonly occur in response to trauma (Stark, 1994; Perls et al., 1951/1976). Despite being strongly resistant to change, because they're unconscious, symbolic visual examples of repetition compulsion can be made by fashioning paper chains, providing an opportunity to finally experience and process what has been hitherto repeatedly defended against.

Each participant creates a mind-map capturing step-by-step actions, feelings, and consequences associated with a trauma narrative, and each step is turned into a link. The links are then chained together in the order in which they occurred, and additional links are added to connect up feelings, actions, or behaviours that are re-occurring. The tangled 3D visual sculptures which result, are then discussed with the group, who support and witness each participant make one cut, releasing some links, which then become accessible to work with (Figure 12.1).

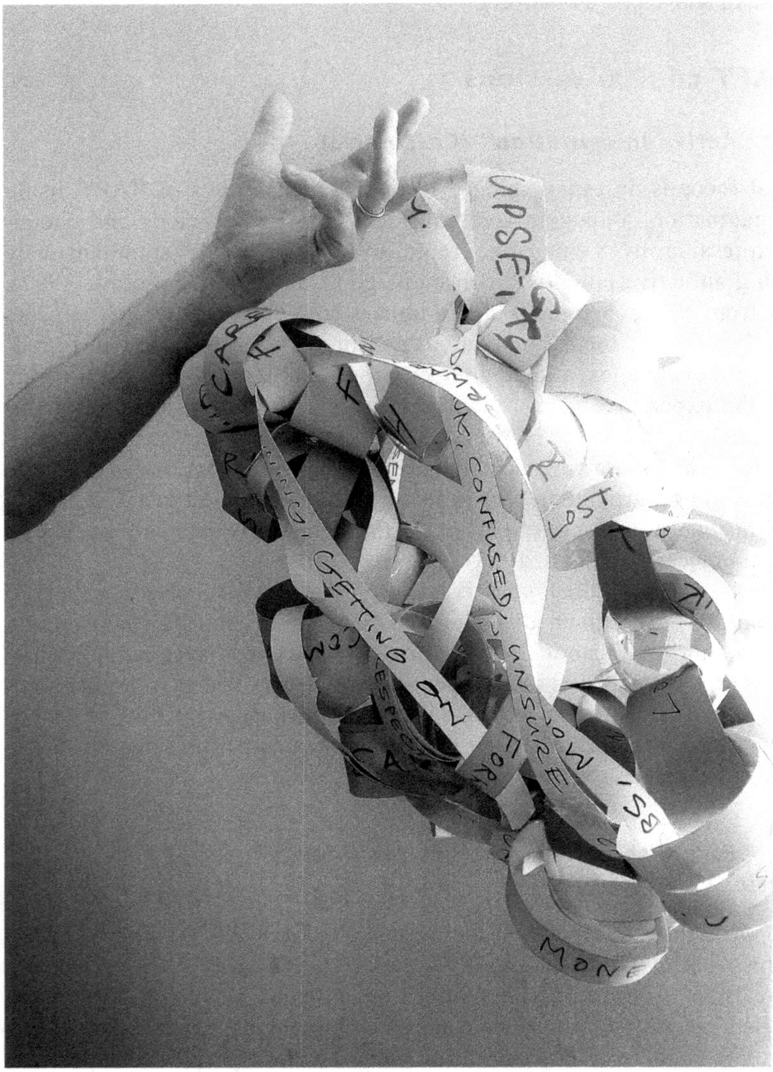

Figure 12.1 Multicoloured paper (orange, green, and white), Sellotape, and marker pen

This intervention reflects the claim that "what is reproduced in a repetition compulsion is what the person needs to feel in order to repair the injury" (Russell, 2006), and the thesis that when there is a need to protect psychological defences, art therapy provides a less threatening means of exploring difficult emotions (Waller and Mahony 1998).

In the companion session, participants draw a large-scale outline of their hand, adding on palm lines, symbolic of *train tracks*, representing their trauma histories. On each *track,* various named *station-stops* are added reflecting their trauma experiences (e.g., *"abuse-alley"* or *"addiction-avenue"*). Each fingertip symbolises a desired destination, goal, or treatment outcome. *Train* lines are then added down each finger, to connect up with the *tracks* on the palm. Along the length of the finger *tracks*, *station stops* are added, symbolising obstacles which could derail arrival at the desired destinations. The intervention serves as an embodied map, highlighting potential relapse triggers, while simultaneously communicating/affirming that recovery is in their own hands!

Week 3: "Mindfulness and Bodywork" (Conjunctio)

Cultivating mindfulness is beneficial when working with trauma as it provides a pathway to embodiment which is essential to the re-integration of mind and body, a prerequisite of healing. Trauma is routinely dissociated, abetted in addiction by the numbing use of substances. Mindfulness utilises somatic modes of attention that demarcates the ways in which people perceive themselves by differentiating between attention to, and attention with, the body (Csordas, 1993).

The group name aloud the things they see in the room, using vocal and auditory reinforcement which produces a feedback loop, creating an 'orientating response' (Levine, 1997). This is followed by guided meditation based on the elements of air, water, earth, space, and fire, considered to be rudiments of all material existence, including the human mind and body. Attention is then turned to an internal journey through the body, using active imagination to encounter and express feelings in relation to internal spaces, aspects of trauma, invisible scars, wounds, blocks/ barriers, and other somatic/emotional responses to the intervention. Participants then pair up and witness their partner make a body sculpt/pose in response to the active imagination. These shapes are then drawn, life-sized on paper covering the floor, to create a giant interlinked image, representing the collective aspects of trauma, and colour, pattern, words, and symbols individually added, describing the internal landscape experienced in the active imagination.

The second session extends this symbolic coniunctio of mind/body, using Sand play, exploring possible resolutions to trauma inspired by the previous group exercise.

Week 4: "Detoxing Anger" (Putrefactio)

It's been suggested that developmentally anger is not an emotion but a pre-verbal, pre-cognitive coping mechanism, functioning to ensure the infants physical and psychic survival, when they are at their most vulnerable (Parker-Hall, 2009). In relation to attachment theory, the psyche's *"self-care system"* (Kalsched 1996) can be thought of as a set of internal working models reflecting patterns of relationships that have been generalised and internalised (Stern 1985; Knox, 2003). These schemas provide a set of appraisals and expectancies about outer relationships, determining how the interpersonal world is interpreted and experienced.

Anger reactions may be either imploded or exploded. In imploded anger, the breath is held within, creating a gesture of internal collapse/implosion. Untreated, imploded anger can physically result in ulcers, arthritis, and chronic fatigue. There are also secondary reactions identified by Tagar et al. (2018) as sarcasm, cynicism, bitterness, gossip, revengeful actions, and malicious actions. Conversely, in exploded anger, the breath detonates outwardly, usually accompanied by shouting/ screaming, and displays of destruction. Aside from emotional injury, resultant body illnesses associated with this type of anger are high blood pressure, strokes, heart attacks, and inflammatory conditions.

The root of anger is difficult to identify, and consequently many people are defeated by it, but RAFT has adopted a clay intervention, originally developed by Sherwood (2004), combining Jungian Active Imagination with a clay-making-sequence to slow down and highlight the reaction sequence of anger. In doing so, the initial image of wounding is transformed into a dynamic and healing version of the expressed disposition (Henley, 2002).

Week 5: "Dealing with Dissociation" (Coagulatio)

Developing as a result of overwhelming experience that cannot be contained, processed, or reflected upon, dissociation is the means by which survivors of trauma maintain a sense of personal continuity, coherence, and self-integrity by dis-identifying with their bodily experience (Attias and Goodwin, 1999). Philipsson (2001) describes the interruption to contact, which is a result of dissociation, as "splitting into different self-states". Kepner (2001) expresses it as "withdrawal of the energy of awareness, a fleeing from embodied life".

The task of this session then is to support the development of integrative capacity, while simultaneously respecting the creative defensive role of dissociation which needs to be honoured, rather than dismantled. This session supports participants in moving from disconnection to contact, adapted from Frank's bodywork experiencing, "Reaching and Being Reached" (2001).

> Through the rhythms of life, human experience, concerns itself with meeting and being met, influencing and being influenced, reaching and being reached.
> (Frank, 2001: 105)

Each participant plaster-casts their hands in gestural positions representative of their personal traumatic experience (Figure 12.2). The resulting artefacts are collectively positioned to create symbolic visual communications, which are discussed by the group, exploring Jung's (1966: 181) contention that "often the hands know how to solve a riddle with which the intellect has struggled in vain".

Each cast is then *tattooed* inside and out, exploring themes such as vulnerability/emptiness, to support participants to begin tolerating these feelings rather

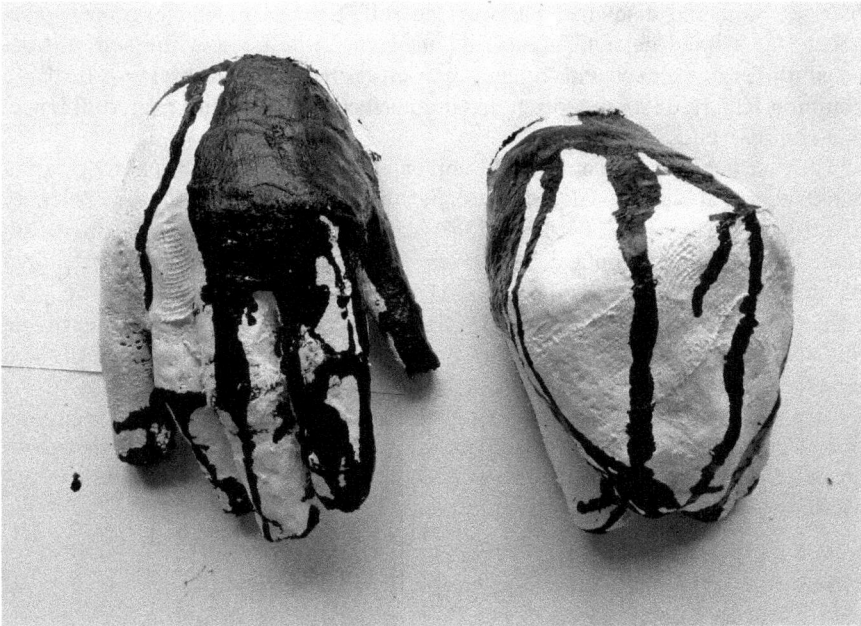

Figure 12.2 Mudroc (plaster bandage) and black acrylic paint

than dissociating, or self-harming. Stern's (2010) work on *'forms of vitality'* further informs the intervention by exploring visually what happens in unscripted speech, when there is something in mind that wants expressing. He posits that "the-something-in-mind" can be an idea, a movement, a gesture, an emotion, a vitality form, or a background feeling, all of which are initially conceived visually, rather than verbally.

Acting as 3D metaphors for healing, the casts also reflect Arnheim's claim that:

> When a metaphor is active it plays with levels of abstraction in order to lay bare a deeper structural affinity between two perceptual images.
>
> (Arnheim, 1969: 138)

Week 6: "Shaking off Shame" (Cibatio)

Shame has been described psychoanalytically as *"the pain of essential unlovability which is beyond speech"* (Wurmser, 1981: 92). In Gestalt terms, Lee and Wheeler (1996) view shame as a rupture between the individual's needs and goals, and their environmental receptivity to those needs and goals, emphasising how shame is a major regulator of the boundary between self and other.

When sufficiently extreme or consistently experienced, *"shame binds"* form as linkages with the disowned parts of the self. Shame thereby becomes internalised as a fixed gestalt, integrated into basic beliefs about the self and the possibilities of contact with others, restricting flexibility. Repression is also a common feature of shame, often driving perfectionism, withdrawal, diffidence, and combativeness.

The first intervention consequently involves giving voice to shame by creating Haiku poems about concealed shame-laden thoughts/experiences/origins, thereby identifying shame binds in order that they can be removed/undone. The poems are shared, stimulating acceptance and compassion, as well as identifying archetypal patterns, combatting the pervasive sense of isolation associated with shame. This reflects the notion that the artwork itself can act as an outlet and holding form that allows the safe externalisation of intense emotions such as shame, anguish, and rage (Johnson, 1990).

The second session involves a collaborative performance exploring the metaphor of the merry-go-round of addiction. Masks created from the poem images are worn to embody individual experiences, before a collective performative unsaddling from the seat of shame takes place.

Week 7: 'Grief/Loss and Psychospiritual Healing' (Sublimatio/Exhaltio)

Kübler-Ross (1969) identified five stages of grief which are also applicable to trauma and addiction. Like alchemy, the stages and process of grieving are not a linear progression, but rather a circumambulation.

The first session incorporates Luigi Zoja's (1989) Jungian philosophy for healing, by embracing ceremony and ritual. Personalising biodegradable sky lanterns or kites, with symbols and words relating to grief and loss, participants take part in a collective letting-go ceremony, designed to rehearse and make possible behavioural changes that support recovery.

In the subsequent session, mandala images are created, using only found materials from nature, reflecting Jung's thesis that a mandala is "the psychological expression of the totality of the self" (1981: 20). The group then visits each mandala in turn, sharing their individual responses, replicating in a group therapy situation the *"interactional process"*, a cooperative creation and an exchange of energy among the three parts: client, artwork, and art therapist (McNiff, 1995).

Week 8: 'Archetypes & Onward Journeys' (Projectio)

Attention to endings is particularly significant in RAFT where the withdrawal is from the group, therapist/s, and the Therapeutic Community setting. The final week of the programme therefore focuses on onward journeys using ritual to honour the physical separation and celebrate the sacred aspects of progress and healing. Mythologist Joseph Campbell observed in "The Power of Myth" (1989) that "the main theme of ritual is the linking of the individual to a larger morphological structure than that of his own physical body".

In the penultimate session, archetype cards are used to obtain insight into the universal prototypes most active in the psyche, which Jung described as the *"collective unconscious"*. All archetypes manifest in both light and shadow attributes, and participants blind choose three cards they discuss with the group, using collective knowledge to suggest whether the card represents the past, current time, or points to the future.

In the final session, sealed clay *memory pods* are created, containing un-read messages from each RAFT participant and the therapists. These symbolic artefacts protect against relapse long after the group has ended. In the event of a psychological crisis, the pods can be cracked open and the messages read, re-establishing contact with the embodied experiences and safety of the group dynamic, and rekindling the importance of reaching out/re-connecting with others to reduce the sense of isolation that commonly causes relapse.

Conclusion

In this chapter, I have equated addiction with a tumultuous *night sea journey*, one which all too frequently ends in capsize or drowning, otherwise known as relapse. As an integrative art therapist specialising in dual diagnosis, I witness recurring stories from those out of their depth, treading water, or swimming against the tide of addiction, and while there is no rescue for those in peril on the sea, RAFT has become a life-saving buoyancy-aid, supporting navigation to dry land. The unique characteristics of an integrative arts psychotherapy approach, offering multi-art form interventions, and healing across six therapeutic relationship domains, undoubtedly contributed to building the RAFT ark. The first vessel has undergone many refits in dry dock, reflecting feedback from participants, and evidence emerging from an independent evaluation of the programme's efficacy. I am indebted to all those I have worked with who have helped me shape, deliver, and promote RAFT; keeping the alchemical "golden goal" of recovery afloat has been a truly collective endeavour.

References

Albert-Puleo, N. (1980). Modern psychoanalytic art therapy and its application to drug abuse. *The Arts in Psychotherapy*, 7, 43–52.

Arnheim, R. (1969). *Visual Thinking*. University of California Press.

Attias, R., & Goodwin, J. (1999). *Splintered Reflections: Images of the Body in Trauma* (pp. 155–166). Basic Books.

Callaghan, G. (1993). Art therapy with alcoholic families. In D. Linesch (Ed.), *Art Therapy with Families in Crisis* (pp. 69–103). Brunner, Maze.

Campbell, J. (1989). *The Power of Myth*. Doubleday.

Case, C. (2005). *Imagining Animals: Art, Psychotherapy and Primitive States of Mind*. Routledge.

Chodorow, J. (1997). *Jung on Active Imagination*. Princeton University Press.

Clarkson, P., (2003). *The Therapeutic Relationship*. Whurr.

Csordas, T. J. (1993). Somatic modes of attention. *Cultural Anthropology*, 8(2), 135–156.

De Leon, G. (2000). *The Therapeutic Community: Theory, Model, and Method*. Springer Publishing Company.

Flores, P. J. (2007). *Group Psychotherapy With Addicted Populations: An Integration of Twelve-step and Psychodynamic Theory*. Routledge.

Flores, P. J. (2001). Addiction as an attachment disorder: Implications for group therapy. *International Journal Group Psychotherapy*, 51(1: Special issue), 63–81.

Frank, R. (2001). *Body of Awareness*. Gestalt Press.

Gilbert, M., & Orlans, V. (2010). *Integrative Therapy 100 Key Points and Techniques*. Routledge.

Hanes, M. (2017). Road to recovery: Road drawings in a gender-specific residential substance use treatment center. *Art Therapy, Journal of the American Art Therapy Association*, 34(4), 201–208.

Henley, D. (2002). *Clayworks in Art Therapy: Plying the Sacred Circle*. Kingsley.

Herman, J. (1992). *Trauma and Recovery*. Basic Books.

Horay, B. J. (2006). Moving toward gray: Art therapy and ambivalence in substance abuse treatment. *Art Therapy: Journal of the American Art Therapy Association*, 23, 14–22.

Johnson, L. (1990). Perspective creative therapies in the treatment of addictions: The art of transforming shame. *The Arts in Psychotherapy*, 17, 299–308.

Julliard, K. (1995). Increasing chemically dependent patients' belief in Step One through expressive therapy. *American Journal of Art Therapy*, 33(4), 110–119.

Jung, C. G. (1936). *The Psychology of the Transference*. CW 16, par. 455.

Jung, C. G. (1944). *Psychology and Alchemy* (2nd ed. 1968 Collected Works Vol. 12) Routledge.

Jung, C. G. (1934–1954). *The Archetypes and the Collective Unconscious, Collected Works* (1981, 2nd ed., Collected Works Vol. 9, Part 1). Bollingen.

Jung, C. G. (1961). *Personal Letter in Carl Jung and Alcoholics Anonymous*. Ian McCabe, Karnac, 2015.

Jung, C. G. (1966). *Collected Works of C. G. Jung, Vol. 16* (2nd ed.). Princeton University Press.

Jung, C. G. (1968). *The Collected Works of C. G. Jung, Vol. 9, Part 1* (2nd ed., pp. 3–41). Princeton University Press.

Jung, C. G. (1969) [1960]. *The Structure and Dynamics of the Psyche* (Collected Works Vol. 8). Princeton University Press.

Jung, C. G. (1981). *The Archetypes and the Collective Unconscious*. Princeton University Press.

Jung, C. G., & Shamdasani, S. (Ed.). (2009). *The Red Book: Liber Novus*. W. W. Norton & Company.

Kalsched, D. (1996). *The Inner World of Trauma*. Psychology Press.

Kepner, J. I. (2001). *The Highway of Light*. Privately Published Paper by Author.

Khantzian, E. J. (1985). The self-medication hypothesis of addictive disorders. *American Journal Psychiatry*, 142(11), 1259–1264.

Khantzian, E. J. (2012). Perspective reflections on treating addictive disorders: A psychodynamic. *American Journal on Addictions*, 21, 274–279.

Knox, J. (2003). Trauma and defences: Their roots in relationship. *Journal of Analytical Psychology*, 48(2), 207–233.

Kübler-Ross, E. (1969). *On Death and Dying*. Routledge.

Lachman-Chapin (1979). Kohut's theories on narcissism: Implications for art therapy. *American Journal of Art Therapy*, 19, 3–9.

Lee, R., & Wheeler, G. (Eds.). (1996). *The Voice of Shame: Silence and Connection in Psychotherapy*. Jossey-Bass.

Levine, P. (1997). *Waking the Tiger: Healing Trauma*. Atlantic Books.

Mahony, J., & Waller, D. (1992). Art therapy in the treatment of alcohol and drug abuse. In D. Waller & A. Gilroy (Eds.), *Art Therapy: A Handbook*. Open University Press.

Matano, R. A., & Yalom, I. D. (1991). Approaches to chemical dependency: Chemical dependency and interactive group therapy: A synthesis. *International Journal of Group Psychotherapy*, 41(3), 269–293.

McNiff, S. (1988). *Fundamentals of Art Therapy*. Charles C. Thomas.

McNiff, S. (1995). Keeping the studio. *Journal of American Art Therapy*, 12(3), 179–183.

Moon, B. (1994). *Introduction to Art Therapy*. Charles C. Thomas.

Moon, B. (1997). *Art and Soul*. Charles C. Thomas.

Moore, R. W. (1983). Art therapy with substance abusers: A review of the literature. *The Arts in Psychotherapy*, 10, 251–260.

Parker-Hall, S. (2009). *Anger, Rage & Relationship*. Routledge.

Perls, F. S., Hefferline, R. F., & Goodman, P. (1951/1976). *Gestalt Therapy*. Julian Press, Penguin.

Philipsson, P. (2001). *Self in Relation*. Gestalt Journal Press.

Rowland, S., & Weishaus, J. (2021). *Jungian Arts-Based Research and the Nuclear Enchantment of New Mexico*. Routledge.

Russell, P. L. (2006). Trauma, repetition, and affect. *Contemporary Psychoanalysis*, 42(4) Oct, 601–620.

Schwartz-Salant, N. (1995). *Jung on Alchemy*. Routledge.

Sherwood, P. (2004). *The Healing Art of Clay Therapy*. Acer Press.

Shuman, E., Halperin, E., & Reifen Tagar, M. (2018). *Anger as a Catalyst for Change?* Group Processes & Intergroup Relations.

Springham, N. (1998). All things very lovely: Art therapy in a drug and alcohol treatment programme. In *Treatment of Addiction*. Routledge.

Stark, M. (1994). *Working With Resistance*. Jason Aronson.

Stern, D. (1985). *The Interpersonal World of the Infant*. Routledge.

Stern, D. (2010). *Forms of Vitality Exploring Dynamic Experience in Psychology, the Arts, Psychotherapy and Development*. Oxford University Press.

Tagar, M. R., Shuman, E., & Halperin, E. (2018). Anger as a catalyst for change? Incremental beliefs and anger's constructive effects in conflict. *Group Processes & Intergroup Relations*, 21(7), 1092–1106.

Waller, D., & Mahony, J. (1998). *Treatment of Addiction Current Issues for Arts Therapists*. Routledge.

Winnicott, D. W. (1953). Transitional objects and transitional phenomena. *International Journal of Psychoanalysis*, 34, 89–97.

Wurmser, L. (1981). *The Mask of Shame*. Jason Aronson.

Yalom, I. D. (1985). *The Theory and Practice of Group Psychotherapy*. Basic Books.

Zoja, L. (1989). *Drugs, Addiction and Initiation*. Sligo Press.

Part V

Reflections on an integrative approach and innovations in practice

Chapter 13

Collaboration, co-design, and co-production

Perspectives on art as therapy and service user involvement in assessment, treatment planning, evaluation, and research

Daniel Regan, with Claire Louise Vaculik and Jude Smit

Introduction

Over the past three decades, IATE has developed an integrative therapeutic approach that aims to enable practitioners to bring together psychodynamic, behavioural, cognitive, and humanistic theories and all of the arts, using a structural framework that supports a clinician to work sensitively and rigorously across the phases of the therapeutic journey to meet the differing needs of each unique client or group.

We are passionate about empowering and supporting the individuals, families, and communities that we work with to take an active role wherever possible. Working in this way can help a clinician to be creative and to adapt their approach rigorously to best meet a client's needs and therapeutic aims. This approach starts by developing a collaborative working alliance, which encourages shared engagement in the co-design of aims and interventions. It continues across the journey in the grading and pacing of the work as this unfolds, across the six different "relationships" (Gilbert & Orlans, 2010). Later, it encourages reviews of the aims of therapy and can support collaborative evaluation of the work. It is also able to support co-production when undertaking reflections on practice, defined by Springham and Xenophontes (2021, p. 1) as "people who use and provide art therapy services working together to develop theory in such a way that values both the consensus and differences between each perspective".

This chapter provided an opportunity to open up our practice and reflect with an artist colleague, who has experience in using services and who has worked extensively in arts in health. Together, we aimed to consider what might be included in an approach to practice that honours the perspectives of both client and therapist. We wanted to reflect on how differences might be used actively to inform and strengthen the working alliance, questioning power dynamics and moving to a more accepting and collaborative approach. Also, what might be needed in

DOI: 10.4324/9781003155676-19

therapy to support clients and service users to feel "seen" and "met" in the fullness of their intersectional identity and as such, to feel safe enough to explore differences in the therapeutic relationship. In engaging with these issues and wanting to question our own practice, we started a process of shared reflection. This began as a three-way discussion in January 2021 between:

- *Daniel Regan, an artist specialising in exploring complex and difficult emotional experiences, who focuses on the transformational impact of arts on mental health and whose work builds on his own lived experience*
- *Claire Louise Vaculik, an art therapist and gestalt psychotherapist, who has been Director of the IAP training at IATE since 2009*
- *Jude Smit, an integrative arts psychotherapist and Deputy Director of the IAP training since 2020, currently undertaking Psychology Ph.D. research focusing on lived experiences of attempted suicide in Further and Higher Education.*

We hope that this chapter will highlight some of the qualities and approaches that can best support the active involvement of service users across all the stages of therapy and encourage further discussions within the profession.

Service users' voices in art therapy literature

Our work at IATE has been strongly influenced by the history of art therapy and a keen awareness of the advocacy role that was so often present in early practitioners' work. In order to contextualise and frame our discussions and reflections, we explored current literature. We found that although evident in some earlier articles (Turnbull & O'May, 2002; Learmonth & Gibson, 2010; Melliar & Brühka, 2010), the importance of service user voice for research and practice was firmly established in 2011 by Ami Woods and Neil Springham's seminal article, "On learning from being the in-patient". The authors drew upon work by Horvath and Bedi (2002, cited in Woods & Springham, 2011), to remind art therapists that the service user's own judgements about the strength of the alliance are a stronger predictor of therapeutic outcome. In a later article, Springham (2016, p. 113) highlighted the impact of language on practice and research, calling for art therapists "to use language that speaks to all communities involved in art therapy".

Looking at the benefits of service user and dual experience voices for art therapy training and practice, Huet and Holttum (2016) drew attention to the growing importance of engaging with different perspectives. They cited the fact that the HCPC had embedded consultation with service users and carers when updating the Standards for Education, noting that these recognise that "people with 'lived experience' have a positive contribution to make to professional training" (2016, p. 95).

In addition, drawing on work by Johnstone et al. (2018) and Madsen and Gillespie (2014), Chris Wood (2020, p. 151) noted that "mental health work is potentially most effective when it learns from what service-users say and then collaborates with them". Furthermore, she highlighted the value of acceptance, peer support, and clear collaborative communication, which she sees as requiring "a reframing of therapeutic skills". She reflected that this can be challenging for therapists, "because it involves a rebalancing of the relative power in therapeutic relationships" (Wood, 2020, p. 152). She also believes that taking this approach could encourage therapists to look to other cultures to understand these human experiences differently too. Eastwood (2021) considered the impact of white privilege, power, and difference on art therapy as a profession, advocating for "greater consideration of identity markers such as race, gender and class in art therapy practice" (2021, p. 1). She reflected on what taking an intersectional approach might offer art therapy, believing that this could support white art therapists to reflect on white privilege and white fragility and to play a part in addressing structural racism and discrimination in our society.

Springham and Xenophontes (2021, p. 1) noted that co-production invites diversity and participation in the development of theory. They explained how needed this is in the mental health treatment field, which has a "history of power abuse, stigma and exclusion" (2021, p. 1). They highlighted that using this approach "requires flexibility to ensure those contributing lived experience will share control and influence with professionals" (Springham & Xenophontes, 2021, p. 1). Watson et al. (2021) also reflected helpfully on dynamics of power between therapists and service users, noting that power dynamics may well have played a significant role in the issues that have led them to access support. Winter and Coles (2021) addressed this dynamic directly, as a co-authored exploration of the client's experience of art therapy, setting out how the client understood the experience and empowering him to take up his place as an equal.

Exploring enabling factors in therapy from a lived experience perspective

JUDE: You are recognised as a champion for the arts in health and for empowering service user voice through visual narratives. I know that you have spoken openly in many public forums about your lived experience and your work with service users and other professionals who engage in the arts in health sphere to support mental health and well-being.

DANIEL: I do often talk about my experience of being a patient and a client, starting when I was fourteen. I'll be thirty-six soon, so that's quite a long history of services and therapy. I've spent time thinking about the language that clinicians use too and the space between how a doctor or therapist and a patient make meaning. How can we bridge that gap through the language that we use? I have also worked with the arts and mental health for many years and am currently producing a report on diversity and inclusion. For this, I have been exploring ethnic diversity in relation to arts and mental health projects and bringing together all of the themes that come out of the opinion pieces and the case studies of best practice. Many of these seem to carry over into a sort of "best practice" approach for working with people more broadly.

CLAIRE LOUISE: Perhaps we can draw on some of those experiences today too. What different experiences of therapy have you had? What are the qualities in a therapist that enabled engagement for you?

DANIEL: Looking back, two quite different reactions from therapists stand out for me. Both arose in a therapy session, after I had proposed that we use photography as a stimulus for conversation in therapy. I am a photographer and an artist and that's my primary way of recording the world. It's how I think about, how I navigate through, and tether myself to the world.

In the first example, I mentioned to a therapist that it would be really helpful for me to bring printed photographs to the session, because at times it's really difficult for me to start the conversation. Her instant reaction was to refuse, saying: "Absolutely not, that's not what we do here". This was really shocking for me, particularly because of the language she used and the way she abruptly shut down the suggestion. Afterwards, I felt really on guard and invalidated. My way of broaching the subject in therapy was dismissed and not seen as important. It felt like what was important to her was following the structure that she was accustomed to using in therapy. This approach felt completely non-collaborative and it really damaged the therapeutic relationship. After this, I felt that I couldn't trust her and that she had little respect for a key part of my identity. I ended up not pursuing therapy.

In contrast, in the second example, I had a really different and positive experience. I was undertaking eighteen months of intensive psychotherapy, which was a mixture of individual and group therapy. At the time I was also doing a photography Masters course, which was focusing on the impact and benefits of the arts (particularly photography) for people with lived experience of mental health difficulties. I was using my lived experience as the springboard for this. My Masters and the treatment were running in parallel and for me, they overlapped. I mentioned this to my therapist, telling him: "I completely respect that these two things are different – one is my academic research and one is my therapy – but there will be overlaps". I explained that it would be useful for me to bring in photographs, as these would help me to explain and articulate my feelings. I sometimes struggle to remember what has happened over the last week, so I use photography as a way to document things. I have an incredible visual memory, so when I look back at photographs they are really evocative. I can normally tell by the style of the photograph and the way that I've captured it what mood I was in, whom I was with, and where I was. This therapist was completely open to my suggestion and seemed to respect it. He was vulnerable enough to say: "This is unusual and it's not the way that we normally work. I don't know anything about photography, but let's see how we can meet in the middle.

You can use photography, because it helps you to describe how you're feeling and I will be able to get an insight into the way that you think and see the world". Taking such an open, flexible and curious approach made me feel like the therapist had given me the agency to be who I am and also, to make suggestions in sessions. It felt like we were taking a collaborative approach to my care, so that I didn't feel like I was just a cog in that system – I was able to individualise my treatment plan with him. We used this approach throughout the eighteen months and it became a really normal, regular way for us to work.

I think that those two, quite different, responses had such an impact on the way that I was able to engage with treatment. In the first instance, I felt really uncomfortable even going to the building. I would get anxious about waiting for my appointment, because I felt like I was seeing somebody that didn't respect my identity and my individuality. Whereas when seeing the second therapist, I was always excited to go to the hospital and have my treatment. It was something that I actively looked forward to, because I felt like even though the sessions would be very difficult, we had an amazing bond. It was a safe space, where I felt open to exploring things in a way that felt right for me and without judgement. I think that it was because of his openness, his vulnerability and his willingness to say: "this is new for me and let's figure this out together". The other therapist just shut me down straight away, in an abrupt way, and just said, "absolutely not, that is not what we do here". She made me feel so uncomfortable and I just thought, "I don't want to have any kind of openness with this person". I could have handled her professional insecurity, if that is what she was feeling, if she'd just said in a softer way: "I understand what you're saying, but I might need to look into it. Can we talk about it next week?" But that kind of abrupt shutting down made me think, "this is not going to work".

JUDE: The language used is so interesting, as it seems to communicate something of a power dynamic – "That's not what we do here".

DANIEL: Yes, it reminds me of a project that I did working with my medical records, reflecting on that space between clinician and patient and the words used to describe patients. When I accessed my records, I was shocked at the way that I'd been perceived or written about. I became increasingly aware of the distance that there can be between the clinician and the patient. When I looked at my own archive images that correlated to a session and the way that I was feeling, it is obviously completely different to the way in which I'd been recorded by the clinician.

The process helped me to think about how things can get lost and to look at working more collaboratively in therapy, particularly in terms of the language that's used. When I looked at those records I thought, "that's a really insensitive way to describe me, you obviously didn't realise I was going to look at it". This can be quite damaging, so clinicians need to approach note-taking and record-keeping with compassion.

JUDE: Collaboration can be seen as a partnership, a space for us to think together. Could we ask: "How shall we do this? What works for you?" And then perhaps, "How shall we record what we explored today?"

DANIEL: Finding the words together can help. We also need to remember that how one supports people might need to look very different, depending on where someone is from, how they were brought up, or what their culture is. Sometimes clinicians seem to assume that a person can come to a session and engage in a particular way. Or assume that when someone comes to therapy, that they'll be able to find the words to say how they're feeling. This is not true for everyone. I was reading about a culture that doesn't have a word to describe mental anguish – there is a word for physical pain, but the words to describe mental anguish don't exist within that culture. There are other kinds of cultural accessibility issues too, for example, does the session time clash with a call to prayer?

CLAIRE LOUISE: This could have an impact on using the arts in therapy too, because people use materials and imagination so differently. And being creative, using art materials, or what can be represented may be different in different cultures.

DANIEL: We need to think about the many different layers of people's identity and the intersectionality between these, which makes each person so unique. I'm a queer, mixed race person. I don't really fit into the white community, because I'm not white enough. And I don't fit into the black community, because I'm not black enough. If I have a very masculine, white male therapist, it might make me think "that person won't really understand me, because I can't really talk about being from two cultures and being a queer person with them". A therapist doesn't need to know everything about every culture though, if they are able to be open about that and willing to learn. My best experience of being in a therapeutic relationship is when a therapist has been able to say to me: "I don't know what that is, can you explain that to me?" Instead of nodding and pretending, then I ask the question and clearly they don't know what that is at all! Therapist and client both need to be willing to be open to being taught, so that they really listen to each other. For me this is the most important factor in creating a really beautiful kind of synergised relationship, where both of you are working together. That's how I see therapy. It should be collaborative. I appreciate the skills of any professional that I'm working with, but I also want to feel appreciated that I am the expert in my own experience and how I describe things.

CLAIRE LOUISE: At the start of therapy, when one first enters a service there is an assessment, a risk assessment and then a treatment plan starts to develop. What do you think could support collaboration or co-production in those initial stages?

DANIEL: There has been such a difference in my experiences of accessing services. In some, I have had so much more agency to say how I want things to be – the therapist sat down with me and went through things as it if was a conversation, so I was involved. He suggested that we spoke about my experiences and made notes together, so we could think about what felt important for me and what felt important for us. Then we discussed any different goals that we had and chose which to focus on. It was collaborative.

I have found other services really disempowering. A referral into a service can be a slow process and you can become almost passive, as you don't have any power. You write up your form and you wait for people to call you; you have to come in when they tell you to come in. There is the sense that I should feel lucky to even be there, because the wait had been so long and the fight to get there was so tough. Then you can feel like you can't really speak up, you can't use your voice. I've basically been handed a form and just been told, "Fill that out". And the experience of being in the referral process was completely re-traumatising. The way it was set up just dragged all of my trauma up again in an unsupported environment – they sent me forms and I had to write out all the terrible things that happened to me and then put it in a post box.

JUDE: How could you feel met and engaged with, in a way that would support engagement and choice?

DANIEL: The first step for me would be to engage with processes as part of a conversation. Also, I'd like space to be able to draw and respond visually somehow too. After this, we could fill out some of those other types of forms. I need to engage with a human being who outwardly shows compassion and has effective body language. A bit of compassion and a bit of personality can break down that power dynamic. I can see that I'm speaking to someone who is a therapist, so I'm really grateful to be speaking to them, but they're also a human being. Showing that they're here to support me and we're able to go backwards and forwards; there are two people in a room, two people trying to figure this out together, as opposed to it being that hierarchical way of working.

When I've had time-limited therapy offered to me, it has sometimes felt more rigid. I get the sense that I basically have to be better by the end of the timeframe, so that I can be discharged and be a 'success' case. It seems harder for the therapist to be flexible.

In my private therapy though, I have often been able to set the timeline and the goal and this has felt quite different. The therapist seemed able to be more flexible too. Then I don't feel like I'm just another patient number that needs to get churned through the system and be a success.

JUDE: You've highlighted an important tension in the work – who is it for?

DANIEL: Yes. I wouldn't say I'm very goal-oriented, but I often have a fixed point in my mind I would like to reach. Sometimes in therapy, we have had to write down the goal that I wanted to achieve. I remember once getting to the end of the treatment and I hadn't reached any of the goals! For someone like me, who's a perfectionist, this had a really damaging impact. I felt like I'd failed therapy! Which doesn't take into account the kind of flexibility of operating in a world in which things change and events happen. You may not always get to where you thought you were going to get to, because things have changed.

CLAIRE LOUISE: A bit like when moving through dense woodland and you see a clearing ahead. When you get there, the path opens up a bit and you can see further and have more perspective on the landscape. It can look very different than you'd thought, so you need to re-chart your path. If you don't have the space to reflect, reconsider and adjust on the journey, without seeing that process as "failing", it can feel almost like you're not able to travel on the journey that you need to go on. You stick with the original path even though it doesn't lead to where you now think you need to go, perhaps because you both feel like you have to 'succeed' in getting somewhere.

DANIEL: This makes me think of fog, which is so beautiful to photograph. But when you're trying to photograph fog, you think "if I just walk over to that bit I'll get it then. Then when you get there, you're still in it. It just keeps changing and for me, that's kind of a bit like what the therapy journey actually is – it's like, "I just need to get to that bit"; and the whole view changes and you're still in the fog. You can't capture the whole essence of it from any one point, so you can keep moving through it and it looks different as it's changing.

JUDE: Using that metaphor, sometimes it's not about the destination, it is about being on the journey. If you're too focused on the destination and the end point, you may miss the experience – the scenery, the view, and what is around you.

DANIEL: If I'm working with young people on a photography project that's related to mental health, I often bring a whole stack of images that are my visual diary images. We often start looking and I will say to them, "pick a photograph that instantly jumps out at you, don't think about it too much". Then we will start deconstructing it and thinking about if it reminds them of a memory, or why it reminds them of a memory. For example, is it because of what's in the photograph? Or is it how it's photographed? Is it that black and white makes them feel nostalgic? Through this process we start to build up their visual vocabulary and literacy, so that they can start to think about how a photograph makes them feel. I was running a workshop and there was just one photograph that had a human in it. It was a photograph of my mum's hand in hospital, just before she died. Two people picked that photograph and spoke about illness, death and grief and then we built up this narrative of photographs. They had no connection to these photographs and they didn't know the story behind them, but it meant that we had these incredible conversations. I don't think they would have happened if there wasn't a visual element as a catalyst to support having difficult conversations with a stranger. Having something tangible and visual opens up those conversations.

JUDE: This sound like a way of bridging differences too. It reminds me a lot of work that I've done with postcards and sandtray objects in groups. As group members come into the room, they pick two or three and then share what the cards or objects said about how they felt at the time. Or if people don't feel in a place to speak because the emotional pain is too great, they just hold them up. Having the arts or something tangible can serve as a bridge, a shared language, to enable connection.

DANIEL: Going to therapy can be terrifying! Having a conversation is terrifying sometimes too. It's great that people are picking up objects and using them as the starting points for conversations, as it could otherwise feel quite unmanageable and terrifying.

JUDE: Sometimes it can also feel so intolerable or frightening depending on your lived experience of relationships. I worked with somebody who for, I think probably eighteen months of the first part of our work, I'd sit next to, not opposite. We worked out exactly the space that felt right for them, how much distance there needed to be, and eventually, they made the choice that they might like to move slightly more in eyesight line. But again, it was driven by what was comfortable for them.

DANIEL: That's how I see therapy, it should be collaborative. In my work, I have learnt so much from every single person that I've worked with – about the world, about different aspects of it, about myself.

I appreciate the skills of any therapist that I'm working with, but I also want to feel appreciated that I am the expert in my own experience, if there's no collaboration then I think, this isn't going to work.

Conclusions

In reflecting on this discussion that developed over the course of nine months, we noticed that some ideas emerged and then faded, with others gradually taking their place. We later wrote up the material, collated this, and read it through, enabling us to bring different layers to light and to bring some critical thinking to what had emerged. This seemed to deepen and develop the discussion further again. Springham and Xenophontes (2021, p. 3) explain that co-production can be seen "a creative meeting of differentiated perspectives to generate new understanding in such a way that no single contribution dominates". Writing the chapter in this kind of way felt creative and very rich, as we circled around different experiences and different perspectives slowly drawing out the different meanings that we could make of these.

We discovered themes that kept recurring in our discussion: the importance of language and finding ways to bridge the gap between therapist and client through the language that we use; thinking about the use of power in the relationship, so that both parties can take up an active role in shaping the work and experience this as a collaboration; being compassionate in the way we think and write about our client and their experiences; the value of using the client's own language or ways of expressing themselves to meet in a way that they find helpful; being attentive to different perspectives and respectful of culture and difference, starting by being open to not-knowing and to being taught by the other person.

While empowering service users has been fundamental to art therapy practice from the very beginnings of the profession, we know that the theories that we use to make sense of what is happening in the therapeutic relationship have come predominantly from a particular culture, time, and place. We need to be open to making sense of these relationships and the dynamics within them in different ways, using ideas that might emerge from each different perspective and drawing upon theory and research from different countries around the world.

It was also clear from this discussion how important it is for a therapist to be able to question power in the relationship and also, their own ideas about what it means to be the "expert". This can so often be linked to a therapist's feelings of shame about not knowing enough, or not working hard enough for their clients. Instead, what emerged was the value of bringing a grounded, embodied curiosity to our practice and a willingness to venture out into the unknown to explore this terrain carefully with our clients, guided by their lived experience in these places and using our different perspectives to shape this journey step by step as it unfolds.

References

Eastwood, C. (2021) 'White privilege and art therapy in the UK: Are we doing the work?', *International Journal of Art Therapy*, DOI: 10.1080/17454832.2020.1856159

Gilbert, M. & Orlans, V. (2010) *Integrative Therapy: 100 Key Points and Techniques*, London: Routledge.

Huet, V. & Holttum, S. (2016) 'Art therapists with experience of mental distress: Implications for art therapy training and practice', *International Journal of Art Therapy*, 21:3, pp. 95–103.

Johnstone, L., Boyle, M., with, Cromby, J., Dillon, J., Harper, D., Kinderman, P.,. . . Read, J. (2018) *The Power Threat Meaning Framework: Towards the Identification of Patterns in Emotional Distress, Unusual Experiences and Troubled or Troubling Behaviour, as an Alternative to Functional Psychiatric Diagnosis*. Leicester: British Psychological Society.

Learmonth, M. & Gibson, K. (2010) 'Art psychotherapy, disability issues, mental health, trauma and resilience: "Things and people"', *International Journal of Art Therapy*, 15:2, pp. 53–64.

Madsen, W. & Gillespie, K. (2014) *Collaborative Helping: A Strengths Framework for Home-Based Services*. Hoboken, NJ: Wiley.

Melliar, P. & Brühka, A. (2010) 'Round the clock: A therapist's and serviceuser's perspective on the image outside art therapy', *International Journal of Art Therapy*, 15:1, pp. 4–12.

Springham, N. (2016) 'Description as social construction in UK art therapy research', *International Journal of Art Therapy*, 21:3, pp. 104–111.

Springham, N. & Xenophontes, I. (2021) 'Democratising the discourse: Co-production in art therapy practice, research and publication', *International Journal of Art Therapy*, 26:1–2, pp. 1–7.

Turnbull, J. & O'May, F. (2002) ' "GPs' and clients" views of art therapy in an Edinburgh practice', *Inscape*, 7:1, pp. 26–29.

Watson, E., Coles, A. & Jury, H. (2021) 'A space that worked for them: Museum-based art psychotherapy, power dynamics, social inclusion and autonomy', *International Journal of Art Therapy,* 26:4, pp. 137–146.

Winter, N. & Coles, A. (2021) 'The silent intermediary': A co-authored exploration of a client's experience of art psychotherapy for C-PTSD, *International Journal of Art Therapy*, 26:1–2, pp. 29–36.

Woods, A. & Springham, N. (2011) 'On learning from being the in-patient', *International Journal of Art Therapy*, 16:2, pp. 60–68.

Wood, C. (2020) 'Acceptance in the hearing voices movement: How might this be relevant for art therapy service-users?', *International Journal of Art Therapy*, 25:3, pp. 150–158.

Chapter 14

Integrative research
Using art to research art

Gary Nash

Introduction

The importance of incorporating research into practice is recognised as the way in which a new profession generates evidence, develops research methodologies, and adapts practice as new and innovative approaches emerge from clinical experiences. Gilbert and Orlans (2011) consider the integration of research and practice as one of the central principles of an integrative approach so that research informs practice and reflective evaluation of practice informs research. The research component of an integrative arts psychotherapy practice gives a critical framework that supports the practitioner to appraise and develop clinical work in a sensitive, curious, and methodical manner. Research, like creativity, is a way of developing new ideas and testing new methods, this may involve constructing experiments based on the experiences of both client and therapist to further a collaborative understanding of the arts in psychotherapy.

The process of research enables ideas to grow the way an image develops, mark by mark, as themes emerge. Research writing, for me, is like carving and sculpting with words and ideas on the page, as themes develop, come into focus, and crystalise. This chapter will consider what happens when we let visual art making lead the research process.

Art-based research

As reflective practitioners' therapists are constantly studying, reviewing, and critically evaluating what we do in relation to our art-based methods, clinical choices, and collaborative discoveries. This self-reflective learning cycle is described as "reflective practice" in the caring professions (Kolb, 1988; Jones & Joss, 1995) and in a research context, it is known as a "practitioner-research" paradigm (McNiff, 1998a). Using this approach, we study, search, and re-search our practice as we encounter the unique needs and responses of those we work with. Based on the research outcomes, we adapt our methods accordingly. This research approach is grounded in evaluating what we do in order to

DOI: 10.4324/9781003155676-20

understand how we might do it better and is described as "practice-led research and research-led practice" by Waller (2016: p. x). This approach underpins my work, my practice, and all research activities, and is central to an art-based research design.

The term "art-based research" was defined by the pioneering work of McNiff (1993, 1998a, 2008, 2013). The approach described in *Art-Based Research* (1998a) established a clear position in relation to research and the centrality of the creative experience at the heart of art therapy practice. McNiff's definition includes the integrative and collaborative nature of art-based research:

> Art-based research can be defined as the systematic use of the artistic process, and the actual making of artistic expressions in all of the different forms of the arts, as a primary way of understanding and examining experience by both researchers and the people they involve in their studies.
>
> (McNiff, 2008: p. 29)

According to McNiff, artistic expression provides a vitally important way of acquiring and communicating information about human experiences and they underpin our attempts to define what we do as art therapists and as practitioner-researchers. McNiff (1998b) asks us to value art and creative knowledge and use them to extend our creative methods into a formal and systematic study of human experience and phenomena. The 2013 publication of *Art as Research* provides continued expansion of the range of arts media and modalities that are used within therapeutic practice to form the basis of relational and artistic enquiry. The development of art-based research in art therapy in Britain has developed further by Learmouth and Huckvale (2018), Kalmanowitz (2018), and Potash (2018), and in relation to art therapy training and research by Ross (2018), Sinapius (2018), Kossack (2018), and Prior (2018).

The principles of an art-based and integrative research design described by Nash (2021) include: 1) beginning all research with an art form and using an art-based epistemology to expand our knowledge of creative processes; 2) the nature of therapy is relational and therefore requires a collaborative research design involving the intersubjective experiences of all participants, including the practitioner-researcher; 3) the research of art-based processes requires art-based methods of inquiry through which the creative process can be observed, recorded, responded to, and collated. Visual methodologies include a wide range of audio, visual, and digital art forms that document the creative and relational process over time; and 4) an art-based research paradigm moves the focus of enquiry from the art forms of others and what they may reveal – to a focus on the art therapist-researcher's own visual, embodied, and creative responses to the work, the group, or the client–therapist relationship. This places the practitioner-researcher centrally within the research design, giving access to a rich seam of visual and sensory material as we consider the art responses and art-based evidence of the relational work that we engage with.

An integrative approach

An integrative approach to research places the experiences of the researcher-practitioner on an equal footing with the client, their artworks, and subjective experiences of therapy. The relational focus of researching therapy considers the therapist's subjective experiences as being inextricably linked to the implicit and explicit experiences of the client in the therapy relationship. These experiences are seen as a reciprocal exchange of energy, affect, imagery, and imaginative responses that occur in the body and imagination of the therapist and are admissible as evidence and research data. The focus of research therefore places an equal emphasis on the reported experiences of the practitioner-researcher along with the experiences reported by the client, with both participants contributing to a collaborative account.

The creative tension and active agent within the therapeutic relationship are experienced in the intersubjective space between the client and the therapist. The nature of this phenomenon poses considerable problems when we attempt to access verifiable and consistent research data. In verbal therapy, the internal world of both the client and the therapist is accessed through verbal channels of communication and reportage. Coherent data are usually obtained through pre-set questionnaires, outcome questionnaires, statistical analysis of change, reflective summaries, and recorded evaluation reviews or testimonials. In the arts therapies, the intersubjective experiences of both participants are externalised and given form through visual or sensory and arts-based modes of communication. In terms of research, the arts therapies therefore have a range of recorded and replicable forms of subjective information held within the images, movement recordings, sound improvisation, stories, sculptural structures, and poetry created. The creative media and expressive contents form a core part of the relational therapy and can be used as an integral part of an art-based research design.

The questions that concern all research planning is in relation to constructing a research design that uses methods of gathering, as well as methods for interpreting, experiential information, that are congruent with the phenomena being studied. Research into the intersubjective phenomena generated within an integrative arts psychotherapy relationship will need to consider how to access arts objects and recordings, sensory and physiological experiences, and imaginative response material evoked during the therapy. To do this, we need to consider how the body, the imagination, and art are understood as an integral part of the research framework.

Researching intersubjectivity through art

Koch and Fuchs (2011) describe the physical and material experience of arts therapies as being an embodied experience; they propose a theoretical framework for therapists to use based on an understanding of bodily states:

"The body is a particular kind of object. It is the only 'thing' that we can perceive from inside as well as from outside. For this reason, it is intricately related to the problem of consciousness (p. 276). Quoting Merleau-Ponty: "The embodied self is defined by our corporeality (Merleau-Ponty, 1962) or mind-body unity" (p. 277). In their paper *Embodied Arts Therapies*, they define a body-oriented research design to examine the interface between the body, art, and cognition: "embodiment provides a genuine approach to the interface of the arts therapies and cognitive science. It entails the influences of postures and gestures on perception, action, emotion, and cognition" (p. 277). They propose the use of empirical embodiment research that records and documents body movement responses to environmental cues presented through artworks, imagery, postcard, and video imagery. They also consider the importance of working across the arts when conducting research on the therapies. Koch and Fuchs (2011) suggest that

> The knowledge of movement therapy, for example, is well suited to help embodied researchers to better operationalise their body-based interventions and manipulations; the knowledge of music therapy can help better operationalise rhythmic patterns; and the knowledge of arts therapies can help better operationalise the effects of qualia in the visual modality, such as colours or strokes in the use of the body while painting or sculpting.
>
> (p. 278)

A physiological theory of empathy described by Franklin (2010) seeks to understand the importance of the body of the therapist in relation to how we perceive, sense, absorb, and internalise the imagery, words, movements, or sound enactments, made by clients in the arts therapies. Franklin (2010): "In attachment theory, intersubjectivity is defined as the sharing of subjective states with another person through emotional attunement. Similarly, the artist attunes to his or her subject by empathically feeling into the phenomenological object" (p. 160). Franklin combines attachment theory and neuroscience to begin to understand how visual empathy and attunement towards the art of others enables the viewer to feel and imagine the affective experiences of the artist. The basis of his research was to extend this principle and apply it to the art therapist's own visual responses towards the affects experienced, as well as the unspoken dynamic communication, whilst facilitating an art therapy group. Franklin concluded that:

> Art therapists are in a unique position to build on intersubjective understanding by mindfully utilising empathic art to receive, consolidate, and offer back expressions of deflected affect for their clients. In doing so potentially disorganised emotions can be responded to with art and skilful verbal and visual listening.
>
> (p. 166)

Researching art with art

Henzell (1995) introduced the importance of choosing an epistemology that reflects the phenomenon we are studying. He reminds us that research is invariably "to question one's method or purpose or to examine the consequences of one's practice; or to refine or develop it" (Henzell, 1995: p. 190). Henzell considers how research takes many forms and should be tailor made for one's particular purpose by asking: what do you want to find out? Why this and not something else? What is the purpose of the research? And to choose research methods that relate to the type of phenomena being examined. In *Art-Based Research* (1998a), McNiff encourages us to consider an epistemological discourse that includes distinctly artistic ways of understanding such as intuition, imagination, creative expression, and aesthetics. McNiff (2011) argues that research is "a process of disciplined and systematic inquiry where modes of investigation are determined by the nature of the issues being examined" (McNiff, 2011: p. 388).

McNiff (2018) describes the documentation of artistic process and the presentation of research outcomes using examples of art-based methods that seek to observe, witness, and absorb the affective, emotive, and chaotic tensions within the act of image-making. McNiff shows how using art-based methods of observation, participation, imagination, and creative response, we enter into a creative event and experience the sensations triggered by the physicality of art making or witnessing art being made.

These methods include:

- The original artworks along with digital reproductions, close-ups, in-situ, and context
- Digital recording of the image-making process from tripod and forehead mounted video
- Journal entries or sketch books add to the visual narratives and reflective thinking process
- Post-session questionnaires
- Recording of post-session interviews and transcripts
- The artwork made in the sessions forms a part of the reportage
- An edited video is used to present evidence and outcomes.

These art-based research methods seek to take an impression of art-based experiences, from a range of sensory experiential positions, the challenge for the researcher is to formulate a research design that can engage, record, and give access to the subjective phenomenon of creativity in a robust and methodical way.

The methods that we use to collect, collate, and communicate what we witness as practitioner-researchers also include artistic techniques that take an impression of art-based experiences by using similar creative methods that went into making the original artworks. They are based on processes of observing, absorbing, expressing, and recording the practitioner-researcher's creative responses towards the clinical work, imagery, or performance art produced by others. They are described as "response art" by Fish (2012, 2017). Response art is made by the therapist-researcher either before (Gartland, 2012; Fish, 2012, 2013), during a session or group (Franklin, 2010; Satiel & Elliott, 2002), or following a session using post-session impressions and imaginative associations directly expressed through the therapist's "reflect piece imagery" (Nash, 2020).

Response art and reflect piece imagery

Artworks made in relation to clinical work is known generically as "response art", "clinical art", or "counter-transference art" (Moon, 1999; Franklin, 2010; Fish, 2006, 2012, 2017). Fish (2012, 2017) emphasises how response art contains the therapist's experience of clinical material and how the image can be viewed, considered, and examined by the therapist as they are shared and explored further in supervision. The purpose and benefits of response art making are also described as contributing to "self-care, to support with the empathic engagement with clients, and to illuminate countertransference" (Fish, 2012: p. 138). The resulting art works can support the practitioner in areas of self-reflection, self-care, clinical formulation, and research.

In 2018, I decided to formally research this aspect of art therapy practice and the results of the first phase have recently been published (Nash, 2020). The research places the focus of enquiry in relation to post-session response art or "reflect piece" imagery and seeks to gather further evidence of the value and benefits for the practitioner when making clinical art at the end of a session. The aim of the research is to build an evidence base in this area of practice innovation.

Making and reflecting through the image –
a clinical vignette

I will now introduce a series of images to describe how a reflect piece image can emerge and then provide a visual response narrative in supervision. The containing function of the image is an important feature that I use to hold, think about, and engage with my own somatic countertransference in the context described. The sequence of images was made at different times but derive from the same clinical material. *The first image was made at the end of a session and in direct response to a build-up of intense affect, a presence of unprocessed material that I experienced acutely in the body. Figure 14.1 was made with charcoal and eraser. The initial physical movements involved drawing a horizon line across the top of the page and marking five vertical axes that were then shaded, dense at the top of the page, and tapering towards the bottom. The movement on the paper involved a combination of pulling the charcoal towards my body, in particular my stomach, and then cutting across the page from left to right. The charcoal marks are added to by using an eraser to mark vertical highlights from top to bottom and combined with a pivoting torso and vigorous arm movements.*

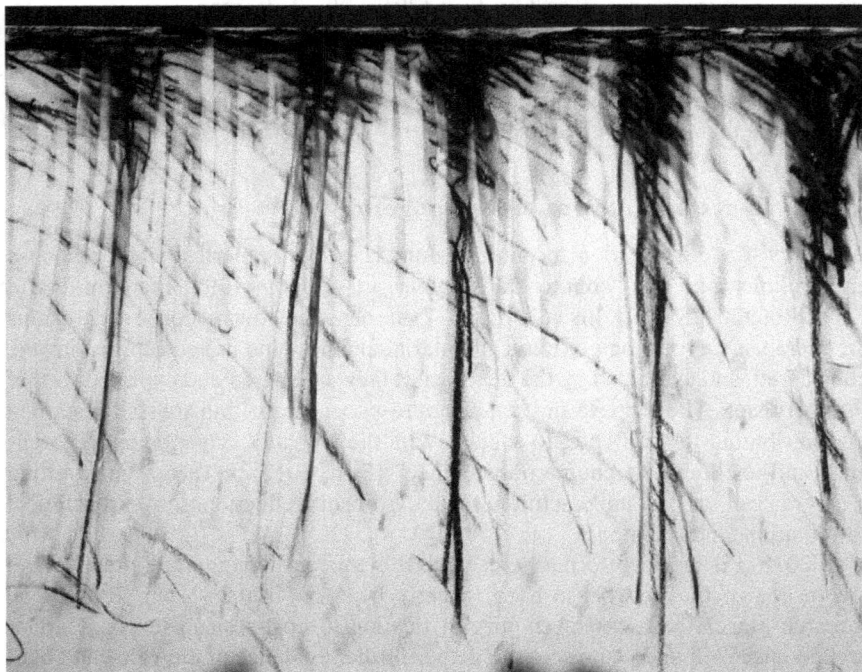

Figure 14.1 Fear in the countertransference. Charcoal and eraser on paper

The image and movement expressed the tension held within my body, a sensation that grew towards the end of a session and which led to an imagined sense of unspoken aggression, hostility, or threat of violence. My immediate feeling was that I was experiencing a persecutory attack and simultaneously a feeling of overwhelming fear, but whether this belonged to me, or the client was unclear and became the focus of supervision. Although not communicated directly, the material was present in the space, palpable, hovering between the client and the therapist, absorbed, and held in my body. When these affects evade processing within the session, the "reflect piece" image provides a visual response that allows this mix of uncertainty, fear, and hostility to be expressed, externalised, and held within the symbolic language of the image.

The memory of the feeling and the image was shared in supervision and enabled me to discuss the affect through the artwork. Reflection in supervision encouraged me to think about the countertransference dimension to the material being presented by the client. My initial response seemed to be evoked by fear of attack and prompted me to consider how that fear may exist in the intersubjective experience of the relationship.

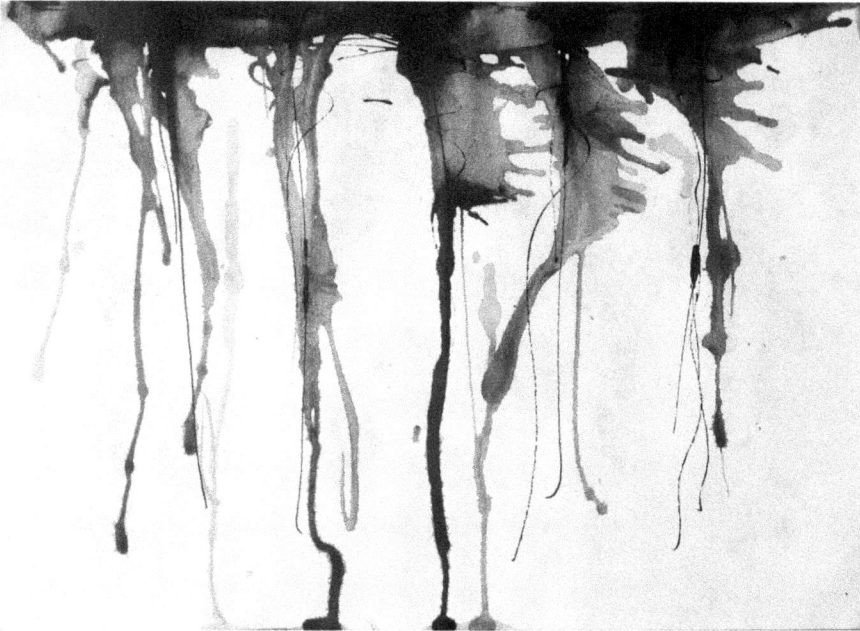

Figure 14.2 Evoking fear. Black ink on paper

I made two further images, one just before supervision began and the third image made in group supervision. In the first image (Figure 14.2), the medium used is ink and the physical enactment enabled me to reconnect with the body memory of the sensations felt at the end of the session. In this image, I found that the way in which the ink stained and dribbled down the page added a "softness", in contrast to the first image, and a deeper, saturated darkness that resonated with the physical feeling across my chest and in my stomach.

The final image (Figure 14.3) was made in a group supervision context, using an integrative arts approach. Before making the image, I experimented with the sound evoked within the embodied feeling. I found that a falling, pouring, tumbling sound, along with the punctuated thud of hitting against the surface of a drum, resonated with the feeling in my stomach and chest. I then made an image that utilised the sound of tearing and ripping combined with elements from the two previous images: the linear structure of the first image with the horizontal axis and the five-pointed vertical lines and the deep, thick liquid medium of the second image. The visceral qualities of the original image are amplified and elaborated through the use of different media and expressive techniques.

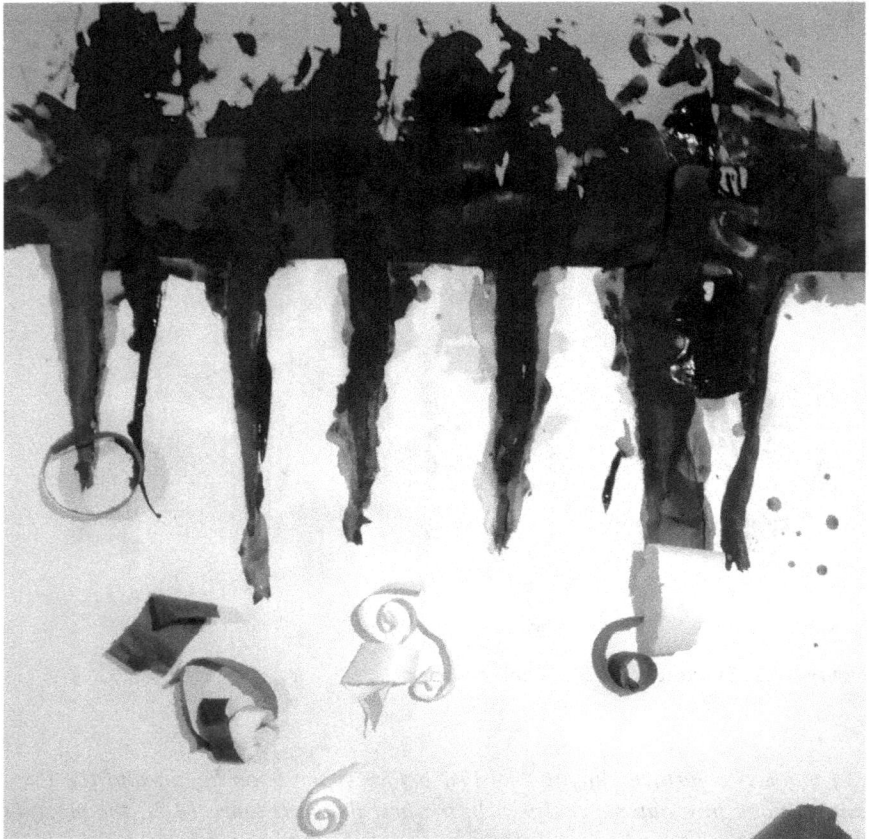

Figure 14.3 Integrating mixed media using sound and torn paper

Viewing all three images in supervision allowed a dialogue to begin in relation to the feelings experienced whilst physically making them. We found that bodily sensations emerged as a reoccurring theme, and I used supervision to examine the quality of each mark/gesture and where it was experienced in the body. The hard, scraping, and rubbing of charcoal, the saturated, soaking, and density of the ink, and the ripping and tearing of paper on paper. These descriptive qualities were derived from the art-making process and then elaborated and extended into metaphors, linking feelings experienced in the body with possible symbolic enactments in the relationship. Images referring to tearing, breaking, and hurting the relationship gave way to pushing away and distancing, which in turn gave way to a sense of withdrawn self-absorption and isolation.

The experience of making a series of images systematically over time shows several processes. First, the memory of the initial feeling that produced the visual metaphor can be re-experienced in the body and bought directly into supervision. Second, as the body memory is bought into the present and mediated through the artwork, so the image can hold and reflect the experience visually, enabling the process to resonate in parallel with the verbal supervisory narrative. The therapist may then re-work the image in response to the exploratory process of supervision, known as "systematic responsive art-making" (Wadeson, 2003). This may involve re-shaping and elaborating the central motif or metaphor as the initial affects are re-experienced and explored in supervision.

The research survey (Nash, 2020) showed that some therapists use this approach to continue to work on response imagery between sessions as they think about and deepen their empathy towards the clinical work and the client being discussed. One interviewee referred to using an *El Duende* or "one-canvas painting" process (Miller, 2012) during systematic response art making. This is a painting method that uses the same image painted and re-painted over an extended period. The image is photographed after each sitting and a gradually changing visual history of the image and the therapist's art-based responses to the therapeutic relationship is digitally recorded.

Response art: mirroring, attunement, and deepening empathy

A new approach described in the research transcripts uses response art to mirror the client's art-making process. This method is described as using the client's remaining palette and sitting in the place where they made art, the therapist uses the same expressive gestures, body movement, and method to recreate a copy of the original artwork. This re-enactment provides a visual mirroring of the creative experience, giving access to a deeper, embodied sense of what it felt like to make a particular image. The experience of immersing fingers into paint and scraping them across, through, and around the page or imitating the vigorous mark-making process can help to find a greater attunement with the client's art expression and non-verbal process. The practice of responding through art and mirroring the expressive gestures seems to support with building empathy and aesthetic attunement (Franklin, 2010) towards what had been described, expressed, or created by the client in the session.

Difficulties and challenges in researching art-based phenomena

Epistemologically research in the arts therapies presents several problems. First, the way images are created is characterised by subjective, non-verifiable, and non-replicable experiences. The source of creativity and the resulting emergence of visual imagery is a process that is "ontologically uncertain" (Hogan & Pink, 2010). Second, the experience of treatment and the benefits gained during any psychological therapy are also subjective, experienced internally, and rely on direct subject-led feedback. The fact that art usually arises from processes that are "interior" to the artist and that therapy focuses on the idiosyncrasies of the individual undergoing treatment (Kaplan, 2001) places the nature of the phenomenon under investigation within subjective and variable parameters that directly impact on research design and methodology.

Using an art-based research design repositions the problem of the subjective nature of creativity and places it at the centre of the research process. The primary position of creative expression within an art-based research paradigm allows art and creative process to capture, record, and generate arts-based evidence in direct response to a creative and relational experience. The researcher can use expressive response art to record internal, and somatic experiences to investigate the intersubjective nature of the therapeutic relationship. Noticing the phenomenological experience in the body and engaging the creativity of the practitioner-researcher brings arts expression into direct relationship with the qualitative content of the subject of research. When a visual arts method is combined with the internal phenomenon of the researcher's subjective experiences of the therapeutic relationship, the art forms can capture a lasting impression of the subjective phenomenon.

The principle of using art and creative expression to research the experience of art and expression within the therapeutic relationship enables us to build visual research methods and to validate and verify their usefulness. We do this by extending the research to capture data from multiple sources. In the research described by Nash (2020, 2021), the practitioner interview and survey questionnaire verified the practice of using response art and validated the experiences and benefits recorded in the research project, notably in the areas of self-supervision and self-care.

Conclusion

The art-based research described in this chapter derives from my art therapy practice and visual arts response to the clinical work. In my experience, the art making continues to enable research to evolve and make unexpected connections between internal physiological experiences and externalised artworks. Thus, capturing something of the imaginal and intersubjective experiences that converge in the creative acts of both therapist and client, in an integrative arts psychotherapy session. Response art places the art of the therapist at the heart of the research design as the therapist responds to the art of others with art. This principle can be extended into any art form as the relational interaction and experience may be given expression through sound improvisation, dramatic movement, sandtray sculp, or other expressive art forms. The range of response art produced may provide a wealth of art-based data in various forms and in different contexts. Each one could form the basis of a study or investigation of the art processes generated "in response" to the clinical work.

If the focus of research is the subjective experiences that occur within the creative and relational space that exists between therapist and client, then the arts therapies have a unique opportunity to use creative phenomena to help us to understand these creative and relational events. In terms of an "embodied research" method described by Koch and Fuchs (2011), response art can channel emotional and physical affects, felt or imagined, into a creative act. The artworks created contain and express a trace of the internal affects experienced by the therapist and are given external form. The inclusion of the therapist-researcher in the inquiry links closely to the phenomena being studied and uses the same dynamic and expressive processes of the arts that we facilitate in our work with others. The resulting artworks provide tangible evidence of some of the intangible experiences that lie at the heart of the arts in psychotherapy.

This chapter contributes to constructing research that is based on the art experiences that form the foundation of art therapy. The research design aims to a) incorporate practitioner-research as a central research paradigm; b) integrate therapists' creative art making into reflective practice that can inform research design; c) elaborate on how art-based methods record a range of dynamic art processes that emerge from creative clinical practice; and d) develop an embodied research framework.

References

Fish, B. (2006) *Image-based narrative inquiry of response art in art therapy*. Doctoral dissertation. Dissertations and theses database (UMI no. AAT3228081). https://www.barbarafisharttherapy.com/publications

Fish, B. (2012) Response art: The art of the art therapists. *Journal of the American Art Therapy Association*, 29 (3), pp. 138–143.

Fish, B. (2013) Painting research: Challenges and opportunities of intimacy and depth. In McNiff, S. (ed.) *Art as research: Opportunities and challenges*, pp. 209–219. Chicago and Bristol: Intellect Ltd.

Fish, B. (2017) *Art-based supervision: Cultivating therapeutic insight through imagery*. New York and Oxon: Routledge.

Franklin, M. (2010) Affect regulation, mirror neurons, and the third hand: Formulating mindful empathic art interventions. *Art Therapy: Journal of the American Art Therapy Association*, 27 (4), pp. 160–167.

Gartland, L. (2012) *Creating space: An exploration into the use of pre-session art-making to process clinical content*. MSc Dissertation, University of East London, London.

Gilbert, M. & Orlans, V. (2011) *Integrative therapy: 100 key points and techniques*. Hove, New York: Routledge.

Henzell, J. (1995) Research and the particular: Epistemology in art and psychotherapy. In *Art and music: Therapy and research*, pp. 185–205. London and New York: Routledge.

Hogan, S. & Pink, S. (2010) Routes to interiority: Art therapy and knowing in anthropology. *Visual Anthropology*, 23, pp. 158–174.

Jones, S. & Joss, R. (1995) *Models of professionalism*. London: Jessica Kingsley.

Kalmanowitz, D. (2018) On the seam: Fiction as truth – what can art do? In McNiff, S. (ed.) *Art as research: Opportunities and challenges*, pp. 141–151. Bristol and Chicago: Intellect.

Kaplan, F. (2001) Areas of enquiry for art therapy research. *Art Therapy: Journal of the American Art Therapy Association*, 18:3, pp. 142–147.

Koch, S. & Fuchs, T. (2011) Embodied arts therapies. *The Arts in Psychotherapy*, 38 (4), pp. 276–280. https://doi.org/10.1016/j.aip.2011.08.007

Kolb, D. (1988) The process of experiential learning. In Kolb, D (ed.) *Experience as a source of learning and development*. London: Prentice-Hall.

Kossack, M. (2018) A different way of knowing: Assessment and feedback in art-based research. In Prior, R. (ed.) *Using art as research in learning and teaching*, pp. 61–74. Bristol and Chicago: Intellect.

Learmonth, M. & Huckvale, K. (2018) The feeling of what happens: A reciprocal investigation of inductive and deductive processes in an art experiment. In McNiff, S. (ed.) *Art as research: Opportunities and challenges*, pp. 95–106. Bristol; Chicago: Intellect.

McNiff, S. (1993) The authority of experience. *The Arts in Psychotherapy*, 20, pp. 3–9.

McNiff, S. (1998a) *Art-based research*. London: Jessica Kingsley.

McNiff, S. (1998b) Enlarging the vision of art therapy. *Art Therapy: Journal of the American Art Therapy Association*, 15 (2), pp. 86–92.

McNiff, S. (2008) Art-based research. In *Handbook of the arts in qualitative research*, pp. 29–40. Thousand Oaks, CA: Sage Publications.

McNiff, S. (2011) Artistic expressions as primary modes of inquiry, *British Journal of Guidance & Counselling*, 39 (5), pp. 385–396. DOI: 10.1080/03069885.2011.62

McNiff, S. (2013) *Art as research: Opportunities and challenges*. Bristol and Chicago: Intellect.

McNiff, S. (2018) Doing art-based research: An advising scenario. In Prior, W. (ed.) *Art as research in learning and teaching: Multidisciplinary approaches across the arts*, pp. 79–89. Bristol and Chicago: Intellect.

Merleau-Ponty, M. (1962) *Phenomenology of perception*. London: Routledge.

Miller, A. (2012) Inspired by *El Duende*: One-canvas process painting in art therapy supervision. *Art Therapy: American Journal of Art Therapy*, 29 (4), pp.166–173.

Moon, B. (1999) The tears make me paint: The role of responsive art-making in adolescent art therapy. *Art Therapy: Journal of the American Art Therapy Association*, 16 (2), pp. 78–82.

Nash, G. (2020) Response art in art therapy practice and research with a focus on reflect piece imagery. *International Journal of Art Therapy*, 25 (1), pp. 39–48. https://doi.org/10.1080/17454832.2019.1697307

Nash, G. (2021) The principles of an art-based research design: Response art and art therapy research. In Huet, V. & Kapitan, L. (eds.) *International advances in art therapy research & practice: The emerging picture*. Cambridge: Cambridge Scholars Publishers.

Potash, J.S. (2018) A more complete knowing: The subjective objective partnership. In McNiff, S. (ed.) *Art as research: Opportunities and challenges*, pp. 153–160. Bristol and Chicago: Intellect.

Prior, R. (2018) *Using art as research in learning and teaching*. Bristol, Chicago: Intellect.

Ross, M. (2018) Art as procedure of truth. In Prior, R. (ed.) *Using art as research in learning and teaching*, pp. 15–27. Bristol and Chicago: Intellect.

Satiel, J. & Elliott, L. (2002) State of the art. In Berke, J. et al. (eds.) *Beyond madness*, pp. 147–156.

Sinapius, P. (2018) 'Not sure': The didactics of elusive knowledge. In Prior, R. (ed.) *Using art as research in learning and teaching*, pp. 29–41. Bristol and Chicago: Intellect.

Wadeson, H. (2003) Making art for professional processing. *Journal of American Art Therapy Association*, 20 (4), pp. 208–218.

Waller, D. (2016) Foreword. In Hogan, S. (ed.) *Art therapy theories: A critical introduction*. Oxon and New York: Routledge.

Chapter 15

Creative and collaborative approaches to researching integrative arts psychotherapy

Marie Adams

Creative approaches to research

Therapists are by nature interested in stories. Through the pain and struggle of their own lives, they come to understand and trust the value of the stories they hear from their clients, whether revealed through words, actions, or the arts. There-fore, counsellors and psychotherapists often unknowingly begin their careers as researchers in personal therapy, in collaboration with their therapists. As du Plock (2010) points out, formal, qualitative research is not so different from what we do as therapists within the confines of the therapy room.

The nature of more formal, qualitative research is also collaborative, working with participants in their search for the truth, and meaning, of personal experience. As Eysenck (1976) points out, research need not necessarily be conducted simply in order to prove something, "but rather in the hope of learning something" (p. 9). This chapter focuses on research as an attempt to broaden understanding and give meaning to our own experience through collaboration with others, whether through our work as clinicians or through the more formal avenues of academic inquiry.

This chapter considers therapists' sometimes resistance to research and elabo-rates on the various and embodied experiences of conducting research – the pleas-ure and the pain.

> **AAAAGGGGHHH Research!**
> **A creative approach**

Introduction

I don't believe I've ever begun an introductory workshop to research with trainee therapists when the mood in the room has not been one of dread. Analysing the "data" from the check-in around the room at the beginning of sessions, I later began to entitle my workshops "AAAAAGGGHHHHHHHH Research!", which at least provokes laughter and lightens the atmosphere.

Check-ins are important in therapy training, the sharing of "data" concerning each trainee's mood, circumstances, and often their hopes and fears. Research

DOI: 10.4324/9781003155676-21

is also fundamental to our work as therapists. From the moment we ask a client their name, or why they have decided to seek counselling, from the moment we ask them why, or how they believe we may be able to help them, we are conducting research. For all the fear and resistance many therapists feel in relation to research, I wonder how often they consider that they've been collecting "data" all along, including into themselves through personal therapy and supervision? Research at its most basic is nothing more than curiosity acted upon: how, what, where, when, and why.

We can conduct formal, postgraduate, or clinical research, or we can conduct research on a smaller scale for the benefit of our practice, for instance, into a particular aspect of a client's experience, such as abandonment or an eating disorder. Sometimes we read, watch a film, or consult with others to understand an aspect of our own history, thereafter, appreciating better our relationships with others, including our clients. Why is this client triggering this response in me, we might ask ourselves when we feel an unaccountable anger or distaste towards a client? As du Plock (2010, p. 21) points out, our explorations into the history of others are often really an organised attempt at discovering something about ourselves.

In my experience, when encouraging therapists to take up research, there is often a misplaced pre-conception that the process will invariably be "dry", statistically based, and without any creative involvement. By the end of my workshops, what I hope is that the participants will recognise that good research always involves creativity, either in the way an issue or an aspect of life is explored or in the analysis of what has been discovered (the data). What we do with our learning through research can also be creative. Where we publish, or where we distribute or convey our findings, whether we write a pamphlet or a book, present a paper, open discussion groups on a topic with our colleagues, or devise an educational programme, these are all exercises in creativity. What may begin as a simple effort to further our own learning will almost invariably prove helpful to others.

Personal interest

At the age of 40, in the middle of a relatively successful career as a journalist, I decided to train as a counsellor. That decision, so many years ago now, has been my saving grace. However, if I'd known that what began as a humble, three-year diploma course in Person Centred counselling would lead to 20 years of study, culminating in a Doctorate, I'm not sure I would have dared take that first step beyond the safety of the familiar. Curiosity, though, has a way of pulling us in, if only we dare take up the lead and, for every therapist worth their salt, empathic curiosity is their abiding mode of operation. An insatiable curiosity about others, often as an unconscious means to knowing ourselves, is at the heart of our professional approach. As Kottler points out, "Our journey to become therapists began for most of us, not with the urge to save the world or help people, but rather to save ourselves" (2010, p. 2). Certainly, this has been true in my case, and no less so during my doctoral research.

Following a further degree in Integrative psychotherapy, the next leg in my training, I faced a professional complaint. While I like to think I handled this six-month period in my life with some grace and blind faith that I would be exonerated, in truth I was a mess (Adams, 2008). I was afraid and, as Charles and Kennedy (1985) and Ferrell and Price (1993) point out, the anxiety and shame evoked through a professional complaint never quite goes away. This may be where curiosity in my case came into its own. During those awful months in which the complaint was ongoing, several therapists revealed to me troubles of their own, aspects of their personal lives they had otherwise kept hidden. I found this both comforting and a little daunting – how many of us suffer in silence, hiding our distress behind the veneer of our professional persona? This question led directly to my doctoral research. I needed to make some meaning out of my experience, and if I could find some solace in knowing how other therapists were struggling, perhaps others might too.

Research into practitioner/researchers

Counsellors and psychotherapists often find the transition from practitioner to practitioner/researcher difficult, often accompanied by "disorientation, self-doubt and anxiety" (Bager-Charleson et al., 2020, p. 95). As a profession, we are generally "more informed by clinical experience, supervision, personal therapy, and literature than by research findings" (Ibid., p. 96). The fact that much of what we understand as research often reads like dry toast may also be the reason behind many therapists' resistance to beginning formal research. As Bager-Charleson et al. (Ibid., pp. 100–101) point out, many participants in their study claimed the focus of their training was primarily experiential, with very little, and sometimes only token, space given over to learning about research.

Qualitative versus quantitative

My nephew in Canada is on his way to training to become a psychotherapist. First, though, he needs a degree in psychology before he can continue into postgraduate work and move into the more "relational" aspect of his development. In the meantime, he blinds me with statistical language where I sometimes feel as if I've been transported into a somewhat unpleasant alternative universe. I know numbers are important, but they are also not my forte. They can tell me how many people experience one thing or another, but they certainly don't give me any more information about why, or how they came to be considered a particular statistic. This is the difference between qualitative and quantitative research – one gives us the numbers, and the other lets us in on the experience. Both are important, as recent events have indicated.

During the recent pandemic, we were obsessed with the numbers, a collective gasp around the nation when yet another 10,000 people were registered as having died of the virus. We were glued to the television during those five o'clock briefings when the chief medical officer showed us graphs of the virus gathering momentum. The numbers spoke to us, told us the extent of the disaster, and sent hot spikes of adrenaline through our systems for fear of how any one of us might be affected. But we were also intrigued by the stories behind those numbers, the doctors who paid with their lives, the nurses kept away from their children while they cared for patients, and the elderly locked away in care homes without visits from family members. So many people die alone. Research into the impact of the virus on business, the medical system, patient well-being, children, and mental health will be conducted for years to come. Numbers will be crunched, and from those statistics, strategies will be developed on how to move forward. Creativity, we hope, will flourish.

By the time this chapter goes to press, hopefully the Covid-19 virus will be under control. Yet at the time of the first lockdown, the confusion for therapists was profound. How were we to work with clients facing the stress of lockdown, while still adhering to the fundamentals and confidentiality of the therapeutic process? McBeath et al. (2020) were quick off the mark, sending out an online questionnaire (quantitative), with room for comments on the experience of working through this traumatic period (qualitative). The researchers received 335 responses, a huge number considering there is usually a minimal response to online questionnaires. In my view, this was also a statement regarding the need for therapists at the time to be heard and to share their experiences. The findings in this inquiry were significant on both a personal and professional level. Isolated in our therapy rooms, now working remotely, we needed to know how our colleagues were faring. Pretty well, as it turned out, adapting to the new technologies (though not without hiccups), and having to be on the lookout for micro-expressions over sometimes pixelated images of our clients. What was more, 28% of therapists, even this early in the lockdown, could foresee that working remotely would "very likely" become "part of their core service to clients in the future", while another 37% said that this was "quite likely" (McBeath et al., 2020, p. 11). The majority of therapists also stated that, going forward, remote working skills should be a core aspect of psychotherapy training.

Like a sad song that sometimes brings comfort, so in my experience did this research. In McBeath's and his colleagues' curiosity on how the Covid-19 lockdown was impacting their colleagues, they highlighted the need for voices to be heard, and for the profession to change – attitudes towards remote working will certainly have been forced to shift because of the lockdowns.

Qualitative research

For most psychotherapists, qualitative research is often the more satisfying methodological approach as it allows the researcher to explore, rather than proving a point (Eysenck, 1976). The why's and how's of our own lives, and those of our clients, are usually of most interest to relationship-based counsellors and therapists.

One of my favourite books during my investigation into the personal lives of therapists was Robert Coles', The Call of Stories (1989). As a young psychiatrist during the polio epidemic in the 1950s, he found himself writing a series of dry treatise on the "defence mechanisms" of those experiencing the disease (p. 28). After being cajoled by both his wife and his clinical supervisor, he finally saw the light and began writing, instead, the "stories" behind his patients' experiences. In my view, stories are what hold us together as human beings. The stories we tell about ourselves and others are how we make up and understand the world, whether those stories are told through words, pictures, movement, or music. If our understanding of something shifts, so does the story, and vice versa. The whole world of therapy is predicated on this idea; We may not be able to change the past, but we may be able to develop an understanding of our experience. As the story shifts, so might our view of ourselves. We may then begin to approach others differently, allowing them to respond to us in a new way. Again, we re-shape our story to one better suited to who we are, or to whom we may now have become. This process is the essence of creativity, relating stories, re-shaping stories, often most tellingly through the arts, whether through words, pictures, or, as Ackroyd and O'Toole have done, through creating drama (2010).

Tellingly, when working with trainee art therapists focusing on research, towards the end of the two-day seminar, I often ask that they work with a visual image to illustrate their feelings at the beginning of the seminar, leading up to how they feel about the prospect of research now at the end of the workshop. I am always astonished at the degree to which the images are revealing, thankfully usually illustrating a more comfortable relationship with the idea of research at the end! This, perhaps, is my own mini research inquiry, canvassing feedback via a visual medium.

Impact on practice

Through the creative exploration of a client's history, the past is not changed, but the perspective is altered, allowing for choices to emerge in how they respond to others or act in the world. This is not unlike the creativity in qualitative research. Having told ourselves a story, we allow our curiosity to take shape and begin to follow the thread of an inquiry into the experiences of others, in my case how the personal lives of therapists impacted their clinical practice. What I can say with some authority is that because of this research my practice, and the manner in which I conduct myself within it has been impacted in ways I never expected. I have had to consider my own narcissistic qualities – why would any of us think we can even do this job without elements of narcissism running like a ribbon through our psyche? I have also, reluctantly, been forced to acknowledge that I sometimes need a break, rather than ploughing on regardless because "my clients need me", a recurring theme in many of my interviews. And finally, I have had to reflect more deeply on the personal struggles my supervisees and colleagues are facing. During my research, I discovered that, as a profession, we are often judgemental in our attitudes towards colleagues, perhaps as a way of denying our own vulnerability (Adams, 2014). We deny our fellow practitioners the right to suffer like everyone else, despite a running theme during much of our training that we are human, always vulnerable, and perfection is impossible. And isn't it true that in the course of our work with clients, often the deepest changes and insights come about through the discomfort and pain of transference and counter-transference, the enactment of archaic struggles (Mann & Cunningham, 2008)? I believe, like Bager-Charleson et al. (2020), that the greatest learning in research also evolves from the discomfort of the process.

Research as an embodied experience

The Norwegian artist, Edvard Munch (2014) said, "Art grows from joy and sorrow, but mostly sorrow. It grows from human lives".

Research can be painful, heartbreakingly painful. We may start out with an idea, a sense that something of our own experience is of interest, let's say an aspect of childhood trauma, only to discover that despite our theoretical knowledge and the self-awareness so hard won through personal therapy, we are still vulnerable when faced with the depth of what we are now learning about others, and therefore ourselves. Like therapy training, perhaps there should be a warning that research can be a life-changing experience, and not everything will turn out well.

Beginning my research into the private lives of therapists, I had no idea how I would be impacted, both emotionally and physically. Over the course of months, I heard stories of traumatic childhoods, the death of loved ones, psychosis in the family, and the list goes on and on. Following these interviews (40 of them!), I was often left with feelings of desolation and sorrow and, on more than one occasion, I returned to therapy to work out what was being triggered in me, usually a distant echo of archaic experience.

In the cohort of doctoral candidates with whom I am currently working, aspects of therapy practice being explored include: using the visual arts to explore adverse childhood experiences and agency, and an exploration into the therapeutic value of dance and movement. I can reasonably predict now that both these inquiries, deeply personal as they are, will evoke powerful feelings in the researcher at some point during their investigations. As Bager-Charleson and Kasap (2017) point out, emotional entanglement with our subject while conducting research is often a by-product of our inquiry, and may, in fact, be part of our creative data analysis. After all, isn't this what we do in the therapy room, attending to our counter-transferential responses to our clients to better understand their internal processes and their relationship with the world? But what also might be triggered, are historical feelings of pain and disturbance, echoes again of earlier experiences. Creativity exists in how we use that information, how we respond to our clients, and how we use what we know, or are learning about ourselves, to further and deepen our work. As Bager-Charleson and Kasap discovered in their inquiry into the embodied experience of conducting research, the process of immersing ourselves in our findings, or data, is no different. Self-soothing and appropriate self-care are essential in this process, moving away from the inquiry for a time to re-energise and soothe our anxieties about moving forward. Long walks, running, or bicycling are just a few of the simple things we can do to undo some of our frozen thinking. Yoga or meditating, playing the ukulele, or joining a choir are a few others. One participant in a workshop suggested playing the stock market, not something I would find relaxing, but then we are all different and all of us will have our own methods for effective self-soothing. We can only hope that they are healthy, rather than self-defeating. How else are we to care for our clients and research participants unless we take care of ourselves first?

Becoming lost

In her brilliant book, A Field Guide to Getting Lost (2017), the historian Rebecca Solnit argues that becoming lost is an obligation in every worthwhile endeavour:

> It is the job of artists to open doors and invite in prophesies, the unknown, the unfamiliar; it's where their work comes from, although its arrival signals the beginning of the long disciplined process of making it their own.

(p. 5)

There is art in qualitative research, in the creativity of the approach, in the analysis of data in the summarising of conclusions, and of course in the distribution of the findings. But along the way, there is the all-encompassing feeling at times of being completely lost before, as Solnit points out, making the work your own. She also argues that becoming lost, and not knowing where you are going, are two different things (Solnit, 2017).

Supervising therapists/researchers over the years, whether on Masters' degree courses or on doctoral programmes, the process appears the same. There is a point when the researcher is terrified and overwhelmed, unable to think of anything else except the subject under investigation. Completely confused by the "data", the researcher is like someone lost in the forest, moving in circles in the blind hope they will find the path home. Of course, there are times when they also lose hope, and this is often the point when they have the good sense to ask others for support, their supervisor, or their "critical friend", someone less immersed in the work and therefore able take a step back and study the findings with a clear eye. At this point, they may realise they are not so much lost, as simply moving into unfamiliar territory.

In my case, my supervisor was able to point out that among my participants, therapist-parents often pointed out that their clinical work had changed after having children, but only one interviewee spoke of the impact on her work of not having children. As I am a childless therapist, I simply hadn't taken this into account, a significant finding in my view. Every researcher needs others to support them through the process, to help them find their way when they become lost in the overly familiar, or the unfamiliar. As Solnit goes on to point out, "Losing things is about the familiar falling away, getting lost is about the unfamiliar appearing" (2017, p. 22). We may begin our research with an idea that something is true, only to discover that what we have previously believed is only half true, or not the complete picture, or not true at all. In research, we need to be prepared to face the unexpected.

The threat of bias

Personal bias is always a hazard, but again, creativity in our approach can be helpful. I remember writing my notes following a particularly uncomfortable research interview which I believed was a disaster. The participant had expressed a belief that our personal lives do impact our work, but he couldn't see how his own work was impacted. No matter how hard I worked at trying to delve beneath the surface of his thinking, I failed to evoke anything of his deeper experience, though I did learn that "maybe I drink a little too much", and he sometimes resorted to drugs.

"That was a bad interview!" I declared when I returned home.

"That wasn't a bad interview, Marie", my partner commented, "that's the data".

What I learned from that experience, and the subsequent wise response, was that not every therapist thought like me, or deemed it necessary to consider their experience at a deeper level. At the point of conducting this interview, I now believe I was looking for confirmation of my own beliefs, rather than being open to the views of others, the value of perspectives that differed from mine. This therapist was deserving of support rather than condemnation. This interview also led me to consider therapists' need for self-soothing, the many and varied, healthy or unhealthy ways in which we cope with the pain we face every day in working with clients and which may also trigger personal anxieties. The potential for therapist burnout is not just an idea, it is a fact (Kottler, 2010; Maslach, 1986; Norcross & Guy, 2007).

Creative research in a changing world

Keeping a journal, recording our thoughts and expectations, and the confusion we feel regarding an interview or an emerging theme is fundamental, and not just for keeping a check on biases. Anything that is evoked while conducting our research is of value and worth recording in words or pictures or musical notes, whatever tells the story of our experience. These days researchers have also needed to be creative in their approach, as my supervisee collecting and generating data through the visual arts has discovered. How do you do this on zoom? In her case, she has sent out a packet with basic art materials, such as oil pastels and coloured pens, to each of her online participants. She then invites her participants to create an image in response to the conversational style interview she conducts over the internet. My supervisee also makes observational notes and creates an image of her own, providing one arises in response to the dialogue. She then screen-shots the participant's image and together they discuss the embodied experience of the process and what has emerged. This is an activity of cooperative participation, both researcher and participant are engaged in the data generating process.

My colleague, Sandra Reeve, is a movement teacher and psychotherapist, all her research stemming from what she experiences through movement, her own, and in what she observes and shares with others (2008, 2013). Much of her work is also conducted outdoors. As both Reeve (Ibid) and Ackroyd and O'Toole (2010) illustrate, both the method of conducting research and the manner in which it can be conveyed to the wider profession are a creative process.

Writing up

My colleague, Sofie Bager-Charleson and I, give a course in Creativity in Academic Writing. The course is popular, not necessarily because we are stellar at our jobs, but rather because many therapists appear to be terrified of writing, an essential aspect of formal research, and often informal research too. There is the terror of the blank page, and there is the fear of exposure, as if something of the "imposter" will be revealed. Owning a point of view through writing, opening ourselves up on the printed page seems to me to be a terror sometimes registering only one degree below death, divorce, and speaking in public. There are also self-imposed expectations, for instance, that if something doesn't read well after the first draft, the person is "bad at writing". However, as Anne Lamott points out, there is always the "shitty first draft". She goes on to say, "all good writers write them. This is how they end up with good second drafts and terrific third drafts" (1994, p. 21). I would add that the 10th, 12th, and sometimes 30th draft finally gets us where we want to be. For all fearful potential writers, I advise you to read this book. Reassuring doesn't even begin to describe her affable and brilliant approach.

This, however, doesn't take away from the pain of writing. Like the distress evoked through analysing painful data, so can the writing up of our findings conjure difficult feelings of anxiety. Attempting to tell the truth of someone else's experience through words, usually clicked out on the hard surface of a computer keyboard, is hard work. We cannot simply draw an image of our findings or turn them solely into musical notes. Somewhere along the road, we must use words to elaborate our discoveries, even if our research is based on different art forms.

Thankfully, the discovery that we can all write, that we may need support and may need to take our time, that having flubbed the first draft, this doesn't mean we'll make a mess of our tenth draft, is the joyous conclusion most of our participants express at the end of Sofie's and my workshops. For this, we are eternally grateful, primarily because some pretty good final dissertations have been handed in by people who at the beginning believed they were 'hopeless' writers. Most of them have even gone on to write up their findings for others in books and journals and conference papers. Others have developed training programmes, workshops, and blogs.

And finally . . .

Research matters, whether not only in the more formal inquiries of masters' or doctoral degrees but also in smaller investigations through further reading, visiting art galleries, and/or attending movies or lectures. What we learn and discover and offer for discussion with our colleagues is a way of giving back to our therapeutic community. We help ourselves, but we also extend that help to others through developing knowledge and professionalism. The process can be imaginative and creative, even while being held within the formal demands of dissertations and case studies. The creativity is in our approach to that learning, our openness to new ideas, and a willingness to be challenged in our thinking. I hope that for all of you, becoming lost in your research will open up the world.

References

Ackroyd, J., & O'Toole, J. (Eds.). (2010). *Performing Research*. Trentham Books, Institute of Education Press.

Adams, M. (2008). Abandonment: Enactments from the patient's sadism and the therapist's collusion. In D. Mann & V. Cunningham (Eds.), *The Past in the Present: Therapy Enactment and the Return of Trauma*. Routledge.

Adams, M. (2014). *The Myth of the Untroubled Therapist*. Routledge.

Bager-Charleson, S., & Kasap, Z. (2017). Embodied situatedness and emotional entanglement in research – an autoethnographic hybrid inquiry into the experience of doing data analysis. *Counselling and Psychotherapy Research*. https://doi.org/10.1002/capr.12122

Bager-Charleson, S., McBeath, A., du Plock, S., & Adams, M. (2020). Becoming a research practitioner: A meta-synthesis. *European Journal for Qualitative Research in Psychotherapy*, 10, 93–109.

Charles, S. C., & Kennedy, E. (1985). *Defendant*. The Free Press.

Coles, R. (1989). *The Call of Stories*. Houghton Mifflin.

du Plock, S. (2010). The vulnerable researcher: Harnessing reflexivity for practice-based qualitative inquiry. In S. Bager-Charleson (Ed.), *Reflective Practice in Counselling and Psychotherapy*. Learning Matters.

Eysenck, H. J. (Ed.). (1976). *Case Studies in Bahaviour Therapy*. Routledge.

Ferrell, R. B., & Price, T. R. P. (1993). Effects of malpractice suits on physicians. In J. H. Gold & J. C. Nemiah (Eds.), *Beyond Transference*. American Psychiatric Press Inc.

Kottler, J. A. (2010). *On Being a Therapist*. Jossey-Bass.

Lamott, A. (1994). *Bird by Bird*. Anchor Books.

Mann, D., & Cunningham, V. (Eds.). (2008). *The Past in the Present: Therapy Enactment and the Return of Trauma*. Routledge.

Maslach, C. (1986). Stress, burnout and workaholism. In R. R. Kilburg, P. E. Nathan, & R. W. Thoreson (Eds.), *Professionals in Distress; Issues, Syndromes and Solutions in Psychology*. American Psychological Association.

McBeath, A. G., du Plock, S., & Bager-Charleson, S. (2020). The challenges and experiences of psychotherapists working remotely during the coronavirus* pandemic. *Counselling and Psychotherapy Research*. https://doi.org/10.1002/capr.12326

Munch, E. (2014). *Art Grows from Joy and Sorrow [Plaque on Wall]*. Munch Museum. https://www.munchmuseet.no/en/

Norcross, J. C., & Guy, J. D. (2007). *Leaving It at the Office: A Guide to Psychotherapist Self-Care*. Guilford Press.

Reeve, S. (2008). *The Ecological Body*. University of Exeter.

Reeve, S. (Ed.). (2013). *Body and Performance*. Triararchy Press.

Solnit, R. (2017). *A Field Guide to Getting Lost*. Cannongate.

Index

Note: Page numbers in *italics* indicate a figure on the corresponding page.

For Product Safety Concerns and Information please contact our EU
representative GPSR@taylorandfrancis.com
Taylor & Francis Verlag GmbH, Kaufingerstraße 24, 80331 München, Germany